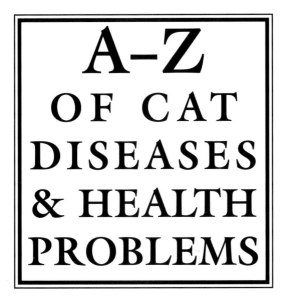

A–Z
OF CAT
DISEASES
& HEALTH
PROBLEMS

Signs • Diagnoses • Causes
Treatment

Bradley Viner
BVet Med MRCVS

HOWELL
BOOK
HOUSE

Howell Book House
New York

636.8089
Vin

Copyright © 1998 by Ringpress Books.

All rights reserved including the right of reproduction
in whole or in part in any form.

HOWELL BOOK HOUSE
A Simon & Schuster / Macmillan Company
1633 Broadway
New York, NY 10019

MACMILLAN is a registered trademark of Macmillan,
inc.

Library of Congress Cataloging-in-Publication Data

Viner, Bradley.
 A–Z of Cat diseases & health problems: signs,
 diagnoses, causes, treatment / Bradley Viner
  p.   cm.
 Includes index
 ISBN 0–87605–043–7
 1. Cats – Diseases – Dictionaries.
 2. Cats – Health – Dictionaries
 I. Title
 SF985.V55 1998
 636.8'0896'003--dc21

                                                97–36905
                                                  CIP

Manufactured in Hong Kong

10 9 8 7 6 5 4 3 2 1

CONTENTS

This book is dedicated to my wife, Liz, and my children, Emma and Oliver, for their patience and understanding when they either tried to get me away from the word processor and obtain my attention, or get access to use the computer themselves. I would also like to dedicate the book to my five cats – Claudius, Cattius, Spartapus, Sculley and Mulder, who did their utmost to distract me from writing this book, yet unwittingly provided me with the inspiration that I needed to complete my work.

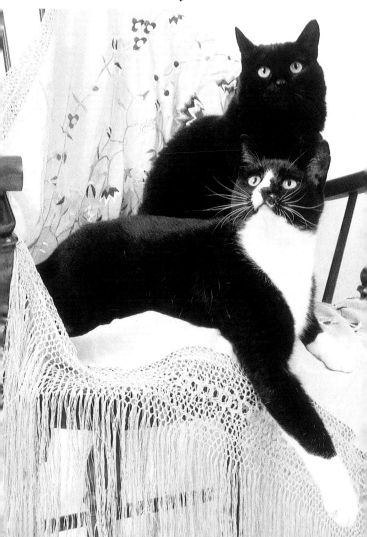

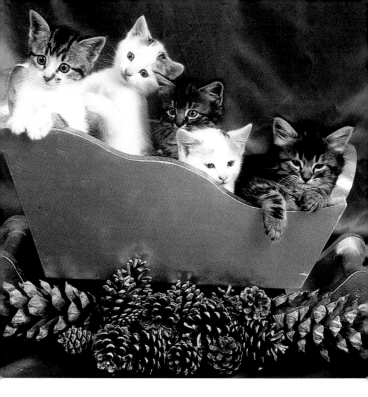

ACKNOWLEDGEMENTS

Grateful thanks to all those who have supplied photographs to illustrate this book, especially to Amanda Bulbeck. Thanks also to Viv Rainsbury for her excellent line drawings.

How To Use
This Book

This book aims to provide the information that the caring cat owner will need in order to keep their cat healthy, to identify problems when they occur, and to gain extra information to supplement the limited amount of facts that can be passed across and assimilated in the stressful environment of a veterinary consulting room. It sets out to provide guidance in an easy-to-understand format with a particular emphasis upon preventative health care, recognising disease symptoms and taking steps to correct them as soon as possible, hopefully before irreparable damage occurs. There is certainly no intention to offer an alternative to a proper clinical examination by a veterinary surgeon.

In Section I, Health and Husbandry, the aim is to give cat owners a better understanding of what makes a healthy cat tick, and how best to care for a cat from kittenhood to old age. The subject of feline behaviour is also examined, helping owners to cope with the behavioural disorders that can sometimes arise when we expect our feline companions to cope with the stresses and strains of living side by side with humans – and often many other cats as well. Situations can arise when some knowledge of first aid could be vital, and expert advice is given on this aspect of cat care. There is also information on nursing a cat when it is unwell, and what to do during the recovery period.

If you are concerned about any abnormal clinical signs that your cat is showing, Section II, Signs of Cat Diseases and Health Problems, provides an easy reference guide. You can look up a sign such as 'Diarrhoea' or 'Thirst, excessive' and be directed to the relevant disease problems that are dealt with in more detail in Section III, Treatment of Diseases and Health Problems. Each sign of ill health is also accompanied by a indicator to tell you how urgently it needs to be attended to.

Section III, the major part of the book, is an alphabetical listing that deals with all of the most important clinical conditions that affect the cat, outlining their clinical signs, causes and treatment. It aims to answer as many of the questions as possible that trouble owners once a diagnosis has been reached and they leave the veterinary consulting room.

SECTION I

HEALTH AND HUSBANDRY

Chapter One

Introducing The Cat

There is no doubt that the domestic cat has turned out to be the pet of the nineties, and is showing every sign of strengthening that role well into the 21st century.

Initially domesticated because of their skill at catching rodents, cats played a vital role in protecting the grain stocks when humans became farmers rather than nomadic gatherers, and consequently cats were revered by the Ancient Egyptians. When a cat died, every member of the family shaved off their eyebrows as a sign of mourning, and the killing of a cat was a crime punishable by death.

CHANGING FORTUNES

The fortune of cats took a major change for the worse in the Western world during the Mediaeval period, when they became associated with sorcery and witchcraft. Cats were publicly burned, buried and even tortured, together with their supposedly satanic owners, to exact a 'confession'. The persecution of the cat allowed a proliferation of rats, very probably playing a part in bringing about the Great Plague which was caused by rats infested with bubonic fleas. This wiped out about a quarter of Europe's human population in just three years between 1347 and 1350 – harsh justice indeed!

The cat was gradually rehabilitated in society

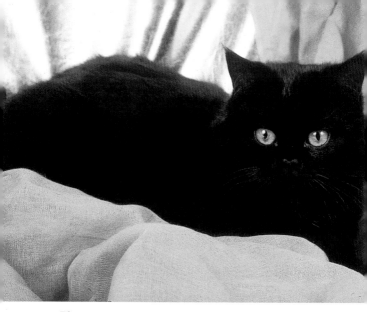

The cat reigns supreme as the most popular of all pets.

through the 17th century; Sir Isaac Newton was a great lover of cats; the diarist Dr Samuel Johnson was devoted to his cat, Hodge, and the poem *The Owl and the Pussycat* was inspired by Edward Lear's cat, Foss. Cats received the Royal seal of approval in this country from Queen Victoria, who owned two blue Persian cats, and working cats played a major role in controlling rodents in factories during the expanding industrialisation of that period.

REIGNING SUPREME

It is only in recent years that the cat has displaced the dog as the number one pet in our affections. Whereas the number of dogs has shown a gradual decline since a peak of just over seven million in the early 1990s, the number of cats kept as pets has steadily increased to well over that figure. It seems that more and more people are finding that the cat fits perfectly into a modern environment, where, in many households, both partners go out to work during the day, and have neither the time nor the space to exercise a pet regularly. Of course, a cat appreciates human companionship (well, most of them do anyway!), but a pair of kittens that grow up together, or an adult cat that has access to the outdoors, can be left on their own more easily while their owners are at work.

Many owners still appreciate the fact that their pet will act as a rodent control officer, although many modern-day cat owners get understandably distressed at their cat's efforts to wipe out the local wildlife population single-handed. Cats seem to catch birds successfully with even the largest of bells attached to their collar, and owners have to console themselves with the thought that predators such as the cat ensure that only the fittest of birds survive, going on to breed further healthy stock. Certainly, most species of garden bird have continued to flourish despite the growing suburban cat population. But the feline's hunting ability is generally low on the list of priorities for modern-day cat owners, and most people choose to live side by side with a cat, for other reasons:

For the elderly, a cat can be a perfect companion.

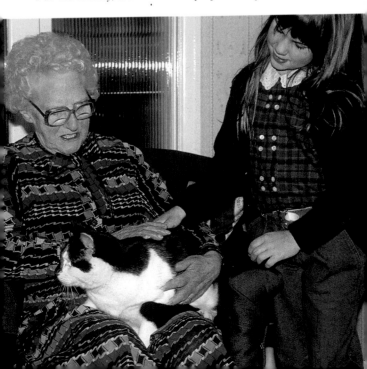

COMPANIONSHIP – we live in an increasingly crowded, yet increasingly lonely, environment, and cats are regarded as close friends by many owners. The loss of a pet cat can affect some people as severely as the loss of a close relative.

EDUCATION – we can learn a lot about the animal world by watching our cats, particularly since they are still so close to nature. The responsibility of helping to care for a pet plays a very useful role in the social development of children. There is considerable evidence to suggest that children who grow up with pet animals become more socially adept and better able to communicate with other people.

HEALTH – while the physical benefit of walking a dog is an added bonus, even the more sedentary activity of owning a cat has been shown to have

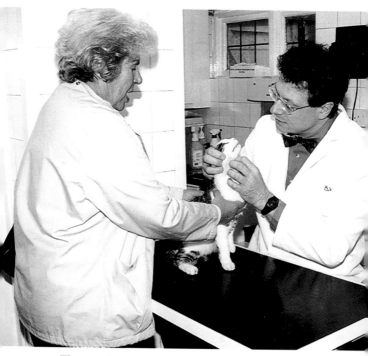

The vet plays an important part in your cat's life.

measurable health benefits. Cat owners have a lower incidence of stress-related illnesses, such as coronary heart disease and strokes, and even take fewer days off work for minor illnesses such as colds and backache. Stroking and caring for a pet reduces stress levels, and this can be measured in terms of lower blood pressure and blood cholesterol levels.

RESPONSIBILITIES

Anyone that makes the decision to own a pet must also accept the responsibility to provide for all of that animal's requirements throughout its life, which, in the case of the cat, can easily extend to sixteen, and sometimes as much as twenty years or more. This will include:-

TIME AND EFFORT – although we have already seen that cats require less attention than dogs, you must still be prepared to dedicate regular time to caring for your cat, especially if it is kept indoors.

FEEDING – the cost of feeding a cat is not great, but they obviously require a high-quality diet fed on a regular basis.

VETERINARY CARE – as well as the routine costs of vaccinations, neutering and other preventative health care, you must be prepared to cope with the unexpected cost of illness or accident. These bills never come at the 'right time' and pet health care insurance is an excellent way of being ready for the unexpected.

BOARDING – many cat owners are able to find a friend or relative to look after their cat when they are away, and a cat that has access to the outdoors can be left for short periods under the supervision of a helpful neighbour. However, a cat should not be left unattended for any length of time, and many owners need to make use of the services of a cattery. This

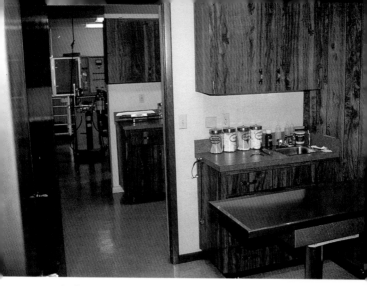

A clean and well-maintained surgery (above). If further tests are needed, samples can be sent to a veterinary laboratory (below).

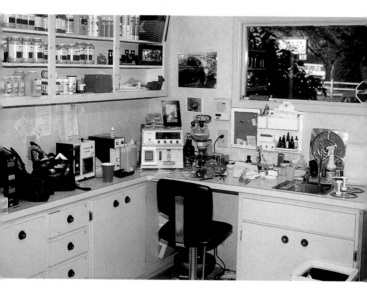

can not only add significantly to the cost of a holiday, but a good cattery will need to be booked well in advance, particularly during the peak holiday seasons.

GROOMING – with many shorthaired cats this is not a problem, as they will take excellent care of their own coat, but many longhaired or elderly cats do require regular grooming. In the case of Persian-type cats, this must be started at a young age and carried out on a very regular basis to prevent knots from forming.

FINDING A VET

Call me biased if you like, but, in my opinion, your veterinary surgeon should play a vital role in the care of your pet, and it is worth building up a good long-term relationship with a surgery in the area, based on mutual trust. Do not assume that you have to be a pet owner before you visit the surgery. The reception staff in a good practice should be willing and eager to give you advice on how to go about obtaining a new cat, and may even know of people in your area with a suitable litter. You should choose a veterinary practice that comes well recommended, looking out for the following points:-

•Waiting and consulting areas should be clean, tidy and odour-free.
•A separate cat waiting area is a great benefit for cat owners and shows the practice is 'tuned in' to the needs of feline patients. There are now an increasing number of 'cat only' practices.
•Polite, friendly and knowledgeable reception and nursing staff.
•Convenient surgery times (often on an appointment basis), and a 24-hour emergency service that does not involve you travelling an unreasonable distance late at night.
•Helpful veterinary surgeons that appear to care for your cat's well-being. Many practices display information about continuing education courses that their members have attended, or additional qualifications that they may have received.
•An effective means of storing your pet's records. Many practices are now computerised.
•A high standard of equipment. Basic facilities should include a well-equipped operating theatre, an

X-ray machine, and adequate hospitalisation facilities. Some may also have on-site laboratory facilities, ultrasound, ECG machines, and many other pieces of high-tech equipment.

Choosing a veterinarian with a high standard of knowledge and care is most important, but this is much harder to judge. Most pet owners feel that, within reason, cost is a subsidiary factor in their choice of veterinary practice, and the prime consideration is to get the quality of care that their cat needs, as and when it is needed.

Chapter Two

THE
HEALTHY CAT

The cat is a killing machine, finely tuned to its function as a dedicated carnivore, hunting at dusk or in the dark for its prey. It is thought to be descended from the African Wild Cat, and many of its physical characteristics still show an adaptation to living in a hot, desert climate. This chapter is aimed at giving the cat-owner an insight into how the body of the cat works, which helps us achieve a greater appreciation of the cat in its normal day-to-day activities, as well as a better understanding of what is happening when things go wrong.

The cat is a mammal, and as such has all of the typical mammalian characteristics:-

WARM-BLOODED: Normal body temperature 38.6 degrees C (101.5F).

HAIRY SKIN: Useful for camouflage as well as temperature regulation.

LIVE YOUNGSTERS: Reared by the mother on milk.

BONY INTERNAL SKELETON: With a basic structure that is shared by all mammals and adapted to their specific needs.

SIGNS OF A HEALTHY CAT

Coat: sleek and glossy

Rear: clean, no evidence of soreness or soiling

Body: lithe and athletic

Ears: clean and pink inside, with no evidence of smell or accumulation of wax

Eyes: clear and bright, free of discharge

Nose: damp to the touch, free of discharge

Mouth and teeth: clean teeth and pale pink gums

THE SKELETAL SYSTEM

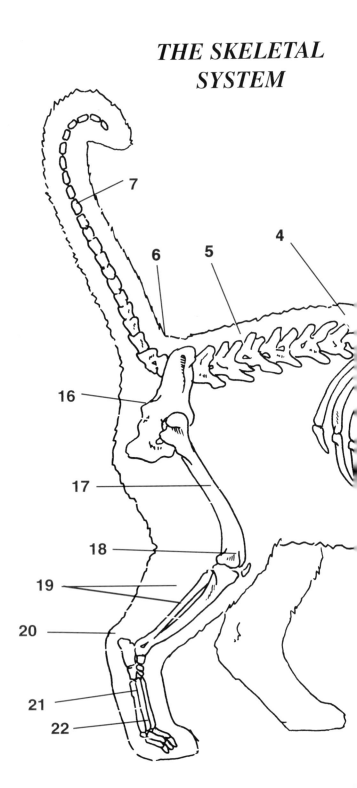

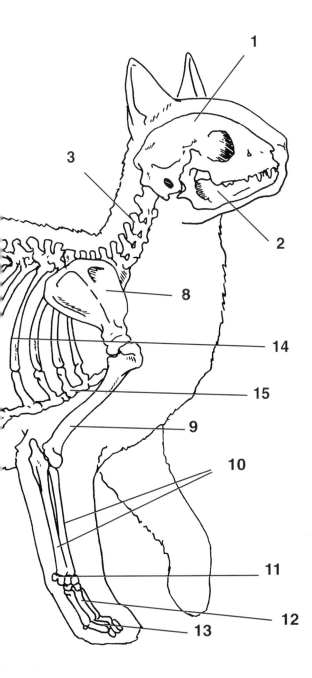

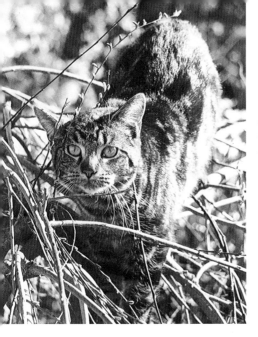

The cat is supremely adapted as a nocturnal hunter.

SKELETON

The skeleton of the cat has about 244 bones, nearly 40 more than the adult human. Most of the extra bones are found in the spine and the tail. The collarbones, or clavicles, are far less developed in the cat than in the human, found just as two very small bones within the muscle tissue or sometimes entirely absent, to allow free movement of the shoulder blade and thus maximum mobility.

The main bones are:

1. CRANIUM: The skull of the cat is smaller in relation to overall body size than in the dog. The bony chamber that is formed by the skull bones is responsible for protecting the soft tissue of the brain from damage, and for containing the scrolled turbinate bones within the nasal chamber, as well as providing attachments for the upper teeth and the powerful jaw muscles. The eyeballs are protected within bony recesses called the orbit, and bones called the zygomatic arches run beneath them to provide further protection from injury.

2. MANDIBLE (or jaw bone): This supports the lower teeth, and is adapted to catching and tearing

apart its prey. It actually consists of two bones joined in the middle of the chin (the mandibular symphysis), and can sometimes split at this site if subjected to severe trauma.

3. CERVICAL VERTEBRAE: Starts start with the atlas and axis, which provide a pivot on which the skull can rotate. Five further cervical vertebrae and their accompanying ligaments provide support and mobility for the neck. Each vertebra is connected to the next by an intervertebral disc, consisting of a fibrous ring with a soft centre that acts as a cushion between the bones. The spinal cord runs from the brain down the bony canal within the vertebral column, carrying nervous impulses in both directions.

4. THORACIC VERTEBRAE: Support the rib cage, with one pair of ribs articulating with each vertebra.

5. LUMBAR VERTEBRAE: Provide attachment for the muscles that form the abdominal cavity wall, as well as those that run along the spine. These help the cat to jump and run, and are articulated in such a way as to allow the cat tremendous flexibility in its spine. This is the most common site of spinal

The cat's spine is amazingly flexible.

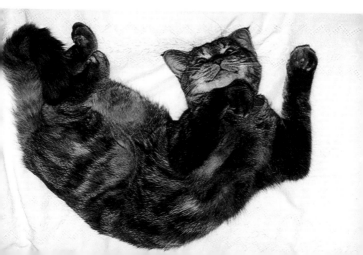

fractures following major injury, which can cause permanent paralysis if the fragile spinal cord within the vertebrae is damaged.

6. SACRAL VERTEBRAE: These are fused together, making a triangular plate of bone that forms part of the pelvic girdle.

7. CAUDAL VERTEBRAE: These form the tiny coccyx at the base of the spine in humans, but in the cat extend along the length of the tail, decreasing in size towards its tip. The spinal cord does not extend down into the tail, which is very mobile, thanks to a complicated system of muscles and tendons that run along its length. The tail is very useful to a cat for balance and communication, but they can cope very adequately without them if necessary. Manx cats are born without tails, or with very short ones, and sometimes have accompanying spinal defects.

8. SCAPULA (or shoulder blade): Provides an important source of attachment for the major muscles of the forearm. It is loosely attached to the body so that it can act like a mobile suspension system, absorbing the shock of impact as the cat jumps. The cat does not have a collar bone like humans, although a tiny trace of them can often be seen in the shoulder muscles on X-rays.

9. HUMERUS: This is a strong bone that attaches the shoulder to the elbow joint. It is covered by the muscles of the forearm, and is relatively well protected from injury.

10. RADIUS AND ULNA: These are paired bones that together form the lower part of the forearm below the elbow. The elbow is a tightly-fitting, hinged joint that only allows movement in one plane. It is not uncommon for one or both of these bones to be fractured, and they often respond well to repair with an external splint such as a plaster cast.

11. CARPUS: This is composed of several bones that together form the equivalent of the human wrist.

12. METACARPAL BONES: These join the carpus to the phalanges. The cat has a fifth dewclaw on the inside of each of its front feet. These seem to play a useful part in the grooming process, with the cat licking them and then using the inside of the fore feet as a sort of comb on its head.

13. PHALANGES: These form the bones of the toe on both the front and hind feet. The cat has retractile claws, which are normally kept withdrawn into a sheath when the cat walks, but can be extended when needed for scratching or climbing. These claws do not wear down on the ground like a dog's, but grow in layers, rather like an onion-skin. When the nail becomes blunt or overgrown, the outer skin is shed, to leave a new, sharp one underneath. It is important that indoor cats are given scratching posts to facilitate this process.

14. RIBS: These surround and protect the chest cavity, and can sometimes be broken as a result of a blunt injury. They articulate with the thoracic vertebrae, and it is the expansion of the chest cavity as the ribs are moved apart that helps to draw air into the lungs as the cat breathes.

15. STERNUM (or breastbone): This joins the ribs together along the lower length of the rib cage. It is relatively soft and cartilaginous, and in some cats, particularly Siamese, the end (xiphisternum) turns outwards to from a small lump that can be felt just in front of the umbilicus or 'belly button'.

16. PELVIS: This is composed of several bones fused together to form a complete ring of bone known as the pelvic girdle. This provides a firm attachment for the large muscles of the hindlimbs, providing the power that the cat needs to achieve its

prodigious jumping capabilities. It is very common for the pelvis to be fractured as a result of a major fall or road traffic accident, although the bones often knit together surprisingly well with conservative treatment in the form of cage rest. Pelvic fractures can cause serious problems during the birth process in entire female cats, or even severe constipation in some cases.

17. FEMUR (or thigh bone): This is the main bone of the hindlimb. The ball-shaped head of the femur articulates with the acetabulum, a socket on the pelvic girdle, and the lower end forms part of the stifle, or knee, joint.

18. PATELLA (or knee cap): This slides on a groove in the femur and helps to keep the knee joint stable. Sometimes the ligament that holds the patella in place may become lax, allowing it to slip out of its normal position in the groove. This can cause the cat to become significantly lame, and may need surgical repair.

19. TIBIA AND FIBULA: Like the radius and ulna in the forelimb, these are paired bones that together make up the lower hindlimb, or shin bone. The tibia is a much larger and stronger bone than the fibula, and runs from the stifle joint down to the tarsus.

20. TARSUS (or hock joint): This is comparable to the ankle joint in humans, and is made up of several bones that articulate with each other. The calcaneus process protrudes from the rear of the hock joint and forms the anchorage point for the large achilles tendon, which acts as a lever to move the lower leg.

21. METATARSALS AND 22. PHALANGES: These make up the hind foot in a similar manner to the bones of the front foot, except the cat has only four digits and no dew claw on the hindlimb.

THE NERVOUS SYSTEM
CENTRAL NERVOUS SYSTEM

This comprises the brain and the spinal cord. The spinal cord is a sealed hollow tube that runs from the brain within the bony vertebral canal down the length of the body. It carries nerve fibres to and from the brain. The cat's brain is protected within the bony skull and weighs 20 to 30 grams (just under one ounce). Although this may seem small, the cat has a higher ratio of brain to body weight than most mammals, other than apes and humans.

The higher centres of the brain, such as the cerebral hemispheres, which are clearly visible as the folded structures on the outside of the brain, are responsible for conscious activities. The cauliflower-like cerebellum behind the cerebrum controls balance, whereas the deeper parts of the brain are concerned with more basic functions such as breathing, instinctive behaviour, and the pituitary gland, which is the 'master gland' at the base of the brain that controls other glands around the body.

BALANCE

The nervous system of the cat is particularly well adapted to allow masterly acts of balance with minimal conscious effort – you have only to watch a cat walk along the top of a wooden garden fence to appreciate this. The nerve fibres are wired in such a way so as to enable the cat to respond extremely quickly to information coming in. The sense of balance originates mainly from the inner ear, where the vestibular apparatus feeds back information to the brain about the position of the head and the motion of the body as a whole.

Perhaps the best known feline 'circus trick' is its ability to land on all fours, even if it starts to fall on its back. A cat does this by using its vestibular apparatus to twist its neck muscles and orientate its head so that it is in a normal horizontal position. It can then jack-knife its body to bring it round into alignment with its head, neatly using its tail to

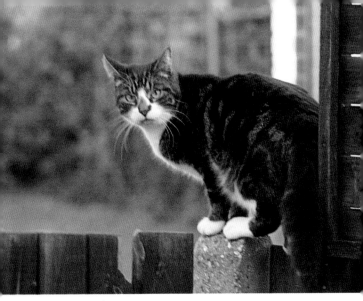

The cat has a masterly sense of balance.

counteract any overbalance that may occur. This righting reflex takes place in a fraction of a second without the need for conscious control.

HEARING

Super-sensitive hearing is essential for an effective night hunter, and the cat is able to hear not only very quiet sounds, but also high frequency sounds that are outside the range of hearing for humans, and even for dogs. This is particularly useful for listening in to the 'conversations' of small rodents and for seeking out the next dinner.

The pinna, or ear flap, is large and cone-shaped, and can be swivelled around towards any distant sounds to collect the slightest sound vibrations. These vibrations are funnelled down the long external ear canal to the eardrum, where three tiny bones, called ear ossicles, transmit the vibrations across the bony chamber of the middle ear and on to the cochlea. This is the actual organ of hearing situated deep in the inner ear, next to the vestibular apparatus.

Cats are not only able to hear very faint or high-pitched sounds, they also have very effective '3D hearing', being able to locate the source of a sound

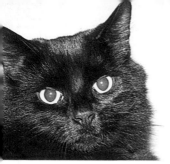
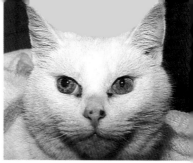

The cat has eyes at the front of its skull, with reflection of light from the back of the eye.

An odd-eyed cat. Difference in colour makes no difference to the cat's ability to see.

very accurately. For example, a cat can distinguish between the source of two sounds just 8 cms (3 inches) apart at a distance of about one metre (3 ft). It does this by being able to accurately compare the time that it takes for the sound to reach one ear compared to the other.

SIGHT

Sight, and particularly night vision, is a highly-developed sense in the cat, and as with most predators, their eyes are large and positioned well to the front of the skull. This means that the cat does not have good all-round vision, and is therefore not able to see anything coming up behind it in the same way as a herbivore such as a rabbit, which has its eyes mounted high up on the side of its skull. This disadvantage is outweighed by the benefit of an overlapping field of vision with both eyes, which gives excellent stereoscopic vision, allowing the cat to judge distances very accurately.

It is not true to say that cats can see in absolute

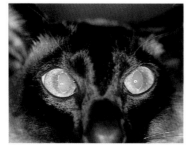

The Siamese squint: This is an inherited condition peculiar to this breed of cat.

darkness, but they are able to see the same details in one sixth of the light that a human needs. This is assisted by the tapetum lucidum, which literally means 'bright carpet', a layer behind the light-sensitive retina at the back of the eye that bounces the light back through the retina and thus magnifies its effect. The pupil is well adapted to functioning at widely differing light levels. Unlike human eyes, the pupil contracts down to a fine vertical slit. The top and bottom eyelids can be closed across the slit horizontally, allowing the cat to let in only a very little light into its highly sensitive eye during the day. At night, the pupil can expand widely to become almost round, and allow in the maximum amount of light. The widely dilated pupil and the reflective layer at the back of the eye is what gives the eerie 'cat's eye' effect – as if the cat's eyes are glowing in the dark.

The retina of any mammal has two types of light-sensitive cells: rods, which are more sensitive in low light but cannot distinguish colour, and cones, which distinguish colour effectively but need good lighting conditions. Cats have about 25 rods to each cone, whereas humans have about four to one, which helps cats to see in the dark, but means that they have very poor colour vision.

The eyelids are responsible for protecting the eye from damage, and maintaining the moist tear film across the surface of the cornea by blinking. The protective function of the lids is augmented in cats by a third eyelid, which can quickly spring across from the inside corner of the eye when danger approaches.

SMELL AND TASTE
As in humans, these senses are closely linked, with smell receptors detecting airborne chemicals and taste receptors on the tongue recognising substances that dissolve in water or saliva. The nasal passages open directly into the back of the mouth, and the overall taste sensation of anything that is eaten will

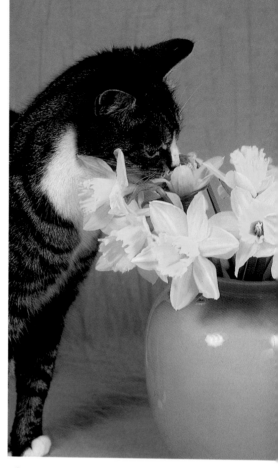

The cat's senses of smell and taste are closely related.

depend strongly upon the sense of smell.

Cats also have a special organ, called Jacobson's organ, situated in a small recess at the back of the mouth that is very sensitive to certain odours, especially those related to sexual behaviour. Cat owners may have noticed their cats, especially entire males, exhibiting a facial gesture termed 'flehmen', in which they hold their head high, their mouth open, and their tongue pressed to the roof of the mouth in order to pass scents on to this specialised scent organ.

Although most mammals respond to sweet, salty, bitter and acidic tastes, cats are unusual because their taste buds show no response to sweet things, but they are very sensitive to the taste of water – one which us humans are unable to specifically detect.

The surface area of the lining of the nose, tightly folded up upon itself within the nasal chamber, is about twice the size of that of a human, despite the smaller relative size of the cat. It is estimated that the sense of smell of the cat is roughly thirty times more sensitive than that of a human, but still relatively poor compared to that of breeds of dog such as the Bloodhound, that have been selectively bred specifically for their tracking skills.

The sense of smell is important to the normal behaviour of the cat, demonstrated by the almost hallucinogenic effect the plant catnip has upon many cats, making them behave as if they are 'high' on drugs. Cats will generally refuse to eat food that they are unable to smell, which can make the nursing of a cat suffering from cat flu very difficult.

TOUCH

Touch is not as important to cats as many of the other senses, but the hairless areas of the nose, the mouth and the paws are particularly sensitive.

The cat's whiskers, or vibrissae, function as specialised organs of touch. They are greatly enlarged and stiffened hairs embedded in the skin of the upper lip to a depth three times greater than that of ordinary hairs. A cat has an average of 24 whiskers, 12 on each side of the nose, arranged in four horizontal rows, and they have strong muscles attached to the base of each hair so that the rows of whiskers can be moved independently. The whiskers

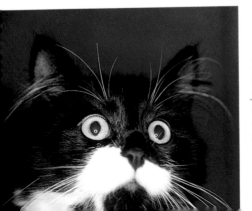

The cat's whiskers function as specialised organs of touch.

are vital for hunting at night, partly to detect any obstacles when navigating in total darkness, partly to detect the movement of air currents, but also to help it kill its prey in the dark.

A cat without whiskers can catch and kill its prey perfectly well in the light, but will plunge its teeth into the wrong part of the prey's body in the dark, and so not kill it cleanly. The whiskers are pulled forward and almost wrap around the body of its prey, reading the shape of it rather like a blind man reading Braille, instantly telling the cat how to react and guiding it to the neck, where its long fangs administer the killing bite.

SKIN

The whole of the cat's body is covered with a protective layer of skin, and its beautiful coat is one of the domestic cat's most striking features. It forms a barrier between the outside world and the cat's inner organs, helping to keep water within the body and protecting against physical injury, extremes of temperature, harmful chemicals, excessive sunlight and dangerous pathogens.

The skin contains several types of glands. Sebaceous glands are associated with the hair follicles, and secrete oily sebum on to the hairs to waterproof them. The sebum also contains special oils that are converted to Vitamin D by the action of sunlight, which is then ingested and utilised when the cat grooms itself. Unlike humans, cats only have

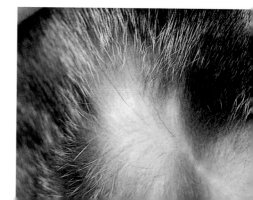

The skin of a healthy cat.

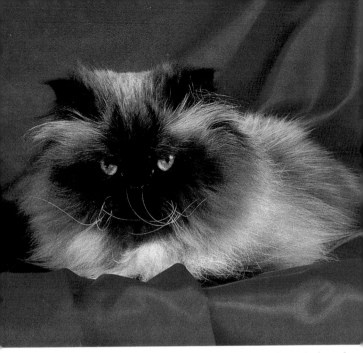

In Longhaired cats, guard hairs may reach 13cms in length.

sweat glands on the footpads, which is why a nervous cat will often leave damp footprints on a veterinary examination table.

Apocrine glands produce a milky secretion that is important as a territory marker, especially on the chin, at the base of the ears, and at the base of the tail. This is why cats will rub the side of their head against familiar objects, and even their owners, marking them with their own special scent.

There are up to 200 hairs per square millimetre of skin, or 130,000 per square inch, with three main hair types:-

DOWN hairs are closest to the skin. They are relatively short, soft and crinkly, providing excellent heat insulation. These are the most numerous type of hair.

AWN hairs form the middle coat, being longer and bristly, with a slight swelling along their length before they thin off at the tip. There are only about one third as many awn hairs as down hairs.

GUARD hairs are the longest and thickest, forming a protective topcoat, keeping the lower hairs dry. For every hundred down hairs, there are only approximately two guard hairs.

The nature of the coat and the relative numbers of the different hairs will vary in pedigree cats. Persian cats, for example, have been bred with very long guard hairs, that may reach 13 cm (5 inches) in length, greatly elongated down hairs, but no awn hairs. The Cornish Rex has no guard hairs and only very short and curly awn and down hairs, and the unusual Sphinx cat has almost no hairs at all!

DIGESTIVE SYSTEM

As a carnivore, the digestive system of the cat is perfectly adapted to catching and killing animals, and then processing meat. This is a much easier task than digesting plant material, and so the length of the digestive tract in the cat is relatively short.

The teeth are designed to catch prey and tear it into pieces – the cat does not chew its food to any extent before swallowing. The adult cat has 30 teeth (two fewer than humans), with 16 in the upper jaw and fourteen in the lower.

The tiny incisor teeth do some ripping and scraping of meat from bone, but are mainly used for grooming.

The large canine teeth are essential for catching and killing prey, slipping between the cervical vertebrae and the skull, dislocating the neck and causing instant death. They have very large roots buried deep into the upper and lower jaw bones.

The premolars and molars have sharp cusps to chop the food into manageable chunks. The last upper premolar is fused with the upper molar tooth, which with the lower molar form the large carnassial teeth, specially adapted for shearing meat and gristle.

The food passes down the oesophagus, or gullet, into the stomach, which is basically a bag where the

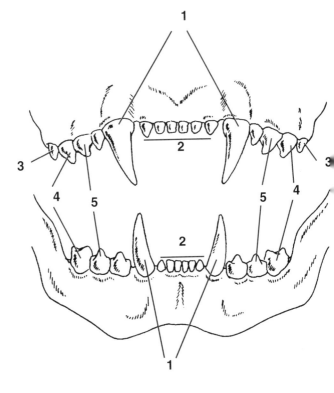

THE CAT'S TEETH

1. Canines
2. Incisors
3. Molars
4. Carnassials
5. Premolars

food is mixed with strong acid and digestive enzymes and stored until it is passed in small amounts on into the small intestine. The main process of digestion takes place in the stomach, aided by enzymes produced by the pancreas and the wall of the small intestine itself, together with bile from the liver. Once it passes into the large intestine, the process of digestion and the absorption of food substances ceases, and excess water is absorbed back into the body. The faecal pellets then pass into the rectum, where they wait patiently (hopefully!) until a convenient moment to be voided.

The cat has become such a specialised hunter that

it has lost certain digestive processes that other animals, even other carnivores such as the dog, still retain. For example, cats have to have a relatively high level of protein in their diet since they have lost the ability to reduce the protein metabolising processes in their liver when protein is in short supply. They also need specific amino acids (the basic building block of proteins) and fatty acids that are only found in animal tissues, whereas other animals are able to alter plant-based amino and fatty acids and to manufacture the full range that they require. For this reason, owners should never attempt to feed cats on a vegetarian diet.

CIRCULATORY AND RESPIRATORY SYSTEMS

The vital organs of circulation and respiration are contained within the thoracic cavity, or chest, protected within the cage of bony ribs and separated from the abdomen by the muscular sheet of the diaphragm. The pleural cavity is a potential space that lies between the lungs and the wall of the chest that is normally only filled with a very small amount of fluid. The two sides of the chest are divided by connective tissue known as the mediastinum, that also surrounds the heart, the oesophagus, and in young animals, the thymus. This is a gland at the base of the neck that is responsible for producing white blood cells in the young animal, but shrivels and all but disappears in the adult.

Air enters the lung through the trachea, or windpipe, and down via the two large bronchial tubes into the smaller bronchi. These tubes are subdivided repeatedly until they end in tiny blind-ended sacs called alveoli. Here, the oxygen diffuses into the bloodstream and the carbon dioxide produced by the body passes into the alveoli to be exhaled. The normal resting respiration rate for a cat is about 40 breaths a minute, about four times that of a human.

The egg-shaped heart lies almost on top of the breastbone, and beats much more rapidly than that of a human – about 120 times a minute at rest, rising to twice that with exercise. Oxygenated blood is returned from the lungs to the larger left side of the heart, where it is pumped around the body in the arteries to the tiny capillaries in the tissues where it is needed. The oxygen is taken out of the blood and the deoxygenated blood is returned in the veins to the right side of the heart, to be pumped back to the lungs again. The oxygen-carrying red blood cells circulate in this double-sided system repeatedly for about a month, and then when they show signs of ageing, they are filtered out by the liver and spleen and replaced with new red blood cells produced mainly in the bone marrow.

The blood also contains several different types of white blood cells involved in protecting the body against attack, such as phagocytes that ingest bacteria and other foreign substances, and lymphocytes that produce antibodies to neutralise pathogens such as viruses. Thrombocytes are small cells in the blood that are essential for the blood-clotting process.

URINARY SYSTEM

The urinary system of the cat is responsible for filtering the blood to remove waste products such as those produced by the breakdown of protein in the body, as well as maintaining the correct balance of water in the body. As the domestic cat was originally a desert-living animal, its kidneys are adapted to carrying out this task very efficiently, and producing only very small quantities of urine when water is in short supply. This is why many owners are concerned by the fact that their cat rarely seems to drink. But cats are able to get most of the moisture that they need from the food that they eat. Absence of thirst is not likely to be of any significance in a cat that is otherwise well, whereas an excessive thirst is a sign that should not be ignored.

Urine is produced by the paired kidneys, which are situated high up in the abdomen, and is passed down the ureters into the bladder. Here it is stored until the bladder contracts and the sphincter muscles relax to push a stream of urine down the urethra to the outside. As we shall see, the anatomy of the lower urinary tract differs considerably between the male and the female.

REPRODUCTIVE SYSTEM

The gonads are glands that produce sex hormones as well as ova in the case of females, and sperm in the case of males. In both instances the gonads start life high up in the abdomen, close to the kidneys, but in the case of the male, the testicles normally migrate via the groin into the scrotum at around the time of birth. Sometimes the testicles remain within the body (see retained testicles page 229).

Eggs produced by one of the two ovaries enter the Fallopian tube, and thence into either the right or left horn of the uterus (womb). Unlike the human, where the uterus has two very small horns and a large body where the two horns join together and the baby normally develops, in the cat the horns are very long and the body short. Because they have so many more offspring in each litter than a human, the foetuses line up along each horn of the uterus rather than in the body. The body of the uterus is normally kept closed by the cervix, or neck, which obviously dilates widely during the birth process. The urethra joins the reproductive tract in the vagina, which then opens to the outside via the vulva, a slit-like opening below the anus.

In the male, sperm produced by the testis are stored in the seminal tubules adjacent to the testicle itself. They can then pass down the spermatic duct and join the urethra just by the prostate gland. This gland is relatively small in the cat, and produces some of the fluid that forms part of the ejaculate when the tom mates with a female. The urethra then passes into the penis, which unlike in many species such as the dog, faces to the rear and is situated just below the scrotum, which is in turn situated below the anus.

The penis of the male is a somewhat fierce instrument armed with barbs, so that intercourse causes considerable pain to the female, which stimulates the ovaries to release the ova. This is called reflex ovulation and is in contrast to the situation in many other species such as the bitch, where the eggs are released from the ovaries on a regular basis regardless of whether mating occurs or not. The urethra of the male is considerably narrower than that of the female, making urinary obstruction a not uncommon condition in the male (see feline urological syndrome page 177).

Chapter Three

PEDIGREE CATS

The vast majority of cats that are kept as pets are non-pedigrees. Many are taken on from friends or neighbours that have bred a litter, others are rescued via welfare organisations, and some just turn up on the doorstep.

The decision to take on a pedigree cat will usually involve more advance planning, and a visit to a breeder to select a suitable kitten. Cat breeds vary much less in size, body shape and conformation than breeds of dog, but nevertheless there are very many breeds and colour variations within those breeds. The decision as to which one to choose is very much one of personal preference, because apart from the need to groom longhaired breeds, there are only minor differences in husbandry between them. This chapter aims to highlight just a few of the more popular breeds and their distinctive characteristics.

PERSIAN

Long-haired cats have lived for centuries in the mountainous regions of Turkey and Iran, but have become extremely popular pets in the last hundred years. At the present time, they are the most popular pedigree cats of all.

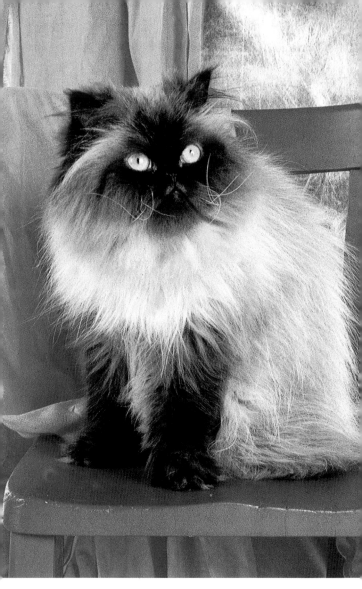

The Colourpoint.

APPEARANCE
As well as a long coat, the Persian has a chunky
body shape, a distinctive round head, and a flattened
face. It has been bred in a wide range of colours,
both self and bi-coloured. They are usually very
placid and laid back cats, ideally suited to an indoors
existence.

TEMPERAMENT
Loving and afectionate, the Persian is a cat with lots
of personality – and they are all very much indiv-
iduals. This is a breed that thrives on human
company.

COAT CARE
The Persian's long coat means that it must be
groomed several times a week. This routine must be
started while the cat is still young, so that it learns to
tolerate, or even enjoy the attention. Once knots are
allowed to form, grooming becomes uncomfortable
or even painful, and the struggle begins.

COLOURPOINT

APPEARANCE
A variation of the Persian cat, the Colourpoint
combines the fluffy body and coat type of the
Persian with the distinctive colouring of the
Siamese. Its eyes are always large, round, and a deep
shade of blue, and the coat is long, thick and soft.

TEMPERAMENT
Coloupoints are generally more lively and vocal
than their Persian counterparts, but they are not
nearly as demanding as a Siamese. Just as with a
Persian cat, regular grooming is essential.

SIAMESE

APPEARANCE
Second most popular breed of cat is the Siamese,
easily recognised by its angular features, elongated
face and limbs, and lithe body. They have a short,
light-coloured coat, which is darker at the 'points' or
extremities of the face, tail and limbs. This is
dependent upon the skin in these areas being at a
lower temperature than over the body itself, and cats
kept in a warm environment will have a darker body
colour. The original Siamese cats were seal point,

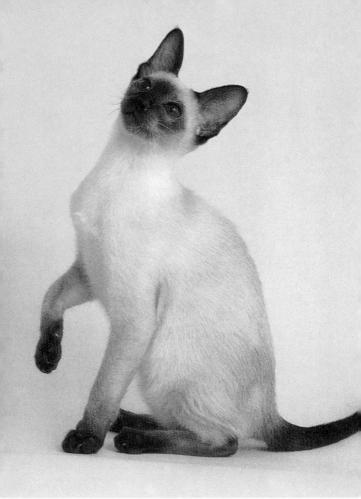

The Siamese.

with a cream coloured body and dark brown points, and although this is still the most common colour, it has been bred in a wide variety of colour variants.

TEMPERAMENT
The Siamese can usually be heard coming from a distance, as it is renowned for its loud and insistent voice. The breed is certainly not for owners looking for a quiet life – a Siamese cat is really a cat-and-a-half, demanding a tremendous amount of attention from its owner, but giving a great deal of love and companionship in return.

BRITISH SHORTHAIR

This breed was developed from domestic non-pedigree cats in the UK during the 19th century.

APPEARANCE

The short coat can be found in a wide variety of colours, although blue is the most common. Despite being quite similar to the domestic non-pedigree cat – and a great deal more expensive to purchase – they are the third most popular breed in the UK. Their body shape is stocky and well-rounded, and the eyes are usually a deep orange.

TEMPERAMENT

The British Shorthair has a gentle and placid nature, making an excellent companion, yet it does not require a great deal of maintenance to keep in good order.

BURMESE

APPEARANCE

The Burmese has a similar 'Oriental' body shape to the Siamese but much less exaggerated, so that the general appearance is of a much more rounded cat. The smooth, glossy coat is a fairly uniform colour across the whole of the body. Brown is the most common colour, but they are found in a five other major colours – blue, chocolate, lilac, red and cream, as well as four tortoiseshell variations of these.

TEMPERAMENT

Like Siamese, Burmese demand a good deal of attention, some of them behaving more like pet dogs than cats. They are lively and sometimes mischievous, and usually love meeting people and investigating new experiences.

RUSSIAN BLUE

APPEARANCE
As the name suggests, the coat of this cat is its main distinguishing feature. It has a unique seal-like texture, and is always a medium shade of blue with an attractive silvery sheen. Even the nose and paw pads are blue, and the almond-shaped eyes are a vivid emerald green.

TEMPERAMENT
The Russian Blue has a gentle and loving temperament, but thrives best in a quiet and secluded environment.

ABYSSINIAN

APPEARANCE
Anyone that has seen the pictures of the cat of Ancient Egypt will recognise the similarity between this breed and their ancient ancestors. Although colour variations have been bred, classically, the Abyssinian has a brown coat colour ticked with black, a slim body, and large ears that ideally have a tuft of hair at their tip.

TEMPERAMENT
Abyssinians are renowned for their friendly and intelligent temperament, and, although not as noisy as the Siamese, they do enjoy a lot of interaction with their owners.

REX

APPEARANCE
There are two separate breeds of Rex cats that have been bred in the UK from mutations that have occurred in domestic cats. The Cornish Rex was developed from just one kitten called Kallibunker that was born in 1950 with a peculiar short, wavy coat and weird, crinkly whiskers. It was bred back to

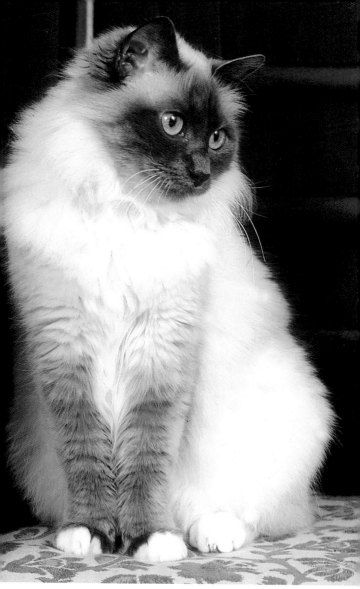

The Birman.

its mother to produce more kittens with the same coat, and has developed into a popular breed that is found in many countries around the world.

The Devon Rex breed was developed from another genetic mutant called Kirlee and was first officially recognised as a breed in 1967. The coat is more tightly twisted than the Cornish Rex. Neither of the

Rex coat types afford very good protection against the extremes of weather.

TEMPERAMENT
Both Cornish and Devon Rex make lively and intelligent pets.

MAINE COONE

APPEARANCE
A long-haired breed that originated in North America that is characterised by a dense, rugged coat that provides excellent protection against the elements and a large, muscular body. They can weigh up to 8kg (18lb) without being excessively fat.

TEMPERAMENT
This breed is ideal for someone looking for a tough, independent, outdoor cat that also enjoys being part of a family when folks are around.

BIRMAN

APPEARANCE
If you see a cat that looks like it has stepped into a tray of white paint, you may well be looking at a Birman. Thought to originate from the sacred temple of cats of Northern Burma, they are a semi long-haired cat with a Siamese coat colouring but with very distinctive white paws.

TEMPERAMENT
They are usually bold cats that enjoy being with people.

COAT CARE
The Birman's coat is easier to care for than that of a Persian or Colourpoint as it is much less prone to matting, but it still needs regular grooming.

Chapter Four

CARING FOR
YOUR CAT

The health care that your cat will require will vary throughout its life, and the aim of this chapter is to look at the different stages of development of the cat and gain an understanding of its needs.

KITTEN CARE
CHOOSING A KITTEN

Having decided that you really do have the making of a suitable cat owner, the first decision that you have to make is to decide if you want to go for a pedigree or a non-pedigree cat. To a large extent this

*If you are looking for a non-pedigree cat,
a private home is a good source.*

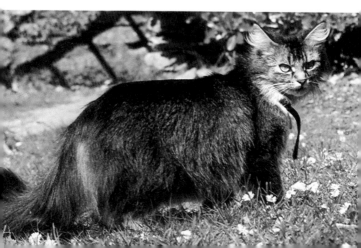

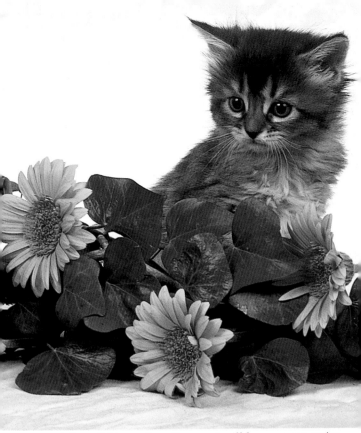

A Somali kitten: A pedigree cat will be more expensive to buy, and could be more costly to keep.

is a matter of personal preference, although a pedigree cat will prove more expensive to purchase, and possibly have higher 'running costs', as they are not always quite as resilient as your average non-pedigree cat.

There are many books that focus on pedigree cats, and for hands-on information about an individual breed of cat, you should consider visiting a cat show in your area to look at the cats and talk to some of the breeders.

If you are after a pedigree cat, and you have decided on the breed, the next step is to look for a reputable breeder. This does not necessarily mean someone that breeds a large number of cats, as a kitten that is reared in an impersonal environment – perhaps in outdoor pens – may not make as well-adjusted a pet as one that has been brought up in the home. You may know of a breeder from other people in your area that have purchased kittens of that particular breed, your vet may be able to recommend someone, or you could look in one of the specialised cat magazines.

Visit the litter in their home, see the environment in which they have been reared, look at the condition and temperament of their mother, and discuss their needs with the breeder. Problems can always arise unexpectedly, but this is the way to get off to the very best start.

If you are looking for a non-pedigree cat, then a private home is a good source. Many pet shops keep a list of litters of kittens available in their area, or your local veterinary surgery may advertise kittens that are ready to leave their mother. Cat rescue centres will often have single kittens or litters that need good homes. The risk of disease may be higher if a kitten has come from an unknown background, but a reputable organisation will check them over carefully before allowing them to leave – and

If you choose two kittens, you will have the pleasure of watching them growing up together and interacting with each other.

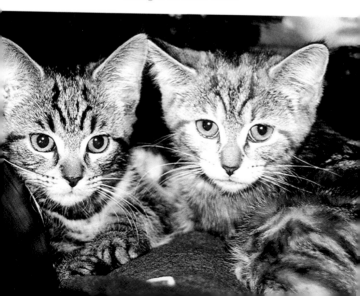

probably check *you* thoroughly as well! It may also be worthwhile considering whether you really do want a kitten, as most rescue centres are crowded with adult cats, which although much more difficult to rehome, often make excellent pets.

It does not make any great difference whether you go for a male or a female, because unless you are planning to breed, either sex will need to be neutered, and both make equally good pets. Some pedigree cat breeders do not allow their kittens to go to new homes until they are twelve weeks of age, but given the choice, it is better to introduce a kitten into its new home as soon as it is fully independent from its mother at around eight weeks.

The final question is whether to go for one kitten or two. It is true that a cat reared on its own may interact more with its owners, but in my opinion, the joy of seeing two kittens growing up together and interacting with each other adds greatly to the pleasures of cat ownership. If the house is to be left empty for a significant part of the day, it is definitely advisable to get two to keep each other company.

GETTING READY

Planning ahead before you pick up your new kitten will help to avoid any last minute panics, but do not go overboard. Basic requirements include:-

CAT CARRIER – don't forget that your little kitten will grow into a much larger cat, so buy a reasonably large one. Plastic or wire-mesh carriers that open at the top are easiest to clean, and the easiest for getting the cat in and out. Avoid wicker baskets at all costs.
LITTER TRAY – large and deep enough to limit the mess, but low enough for your kitten to be able to climb into easily. Some cats feel more secure in a tray with a cover, and some even have a flap for entry and air-vents with deodorising panels to limit the smell!
CAT LITTER – there are many different types, and some cats prefer one to another.

LITTER SCOOP – essential to enable you to clear out soiled litter without delay, and thus greatly assisting hygiene. Most scoops are made up of a coarse mesh to allow the loose litter to fall through and back into the tray again.

FOOD BOWLS – a couple of plastic bowls, one for food and one for water, are fine.

GROOMING IMPLEMENTS – longhaired cats need regular grooming, and you should start as young as possible. A brush tends to skim over the coat, and a fine comb is preferable for preventing knots from forming.

BEDDING – whatever you provide, there is a good chance your new kitten will have its own ideas about sleeping places. Many cats do like to sleep in a secure, enclosed environment, and some very attractive cat beds are available. Your kitten will probably be equally happy with a cardboard box with a hole cut in the front, and you can throw it away and start again when it gets grubby.

TOYS – just as with children, the expensive and sophisticated toys are not always the best, but make sure whatever you do use is safe. Kittens love toys that stimulate their hunting instinct, and a 'mouse on a string' or even just a table-tennis ball can provide hours of fun.

COLLAR – this is important for identification once the kitten starts to go out, although it must have an elasticated section to allow the cat to slip out if it becomes hooked on something.

SCRATCHING POST – important if the kitten is to be kept indoors as it grow up. Elaborate 'cat aerobic' centres are available for the active indoor cat.

FEEDING

Your kitten will have enough changes to cope with at first in a new home, so find out what the kitten is used to eating and stick to it for a few days. Make up your mind what type of food you want to feed in the long run, and gradually change your kitten over to it. The main options are:-

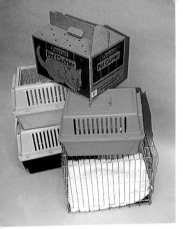

A cat carrier is an essential item of equipment.

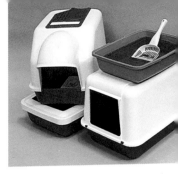

You will need a litter tray and a litter scoop.

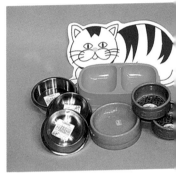

Buy a couple of bowls – one for food and one for water.

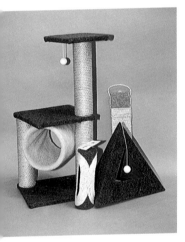

A scratching post is a must if your cat is to be kept indoors.

If you have a longhaired cat, regular grooming is essential.

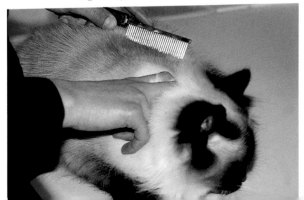

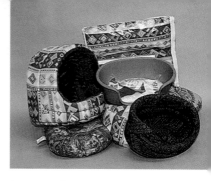

There are lots of different cat beds available.

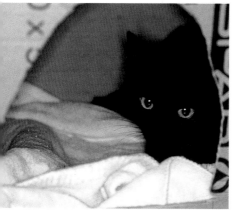

Most cats will be perfectly happy sleeping in a cardboard box with a hole cut in the front.

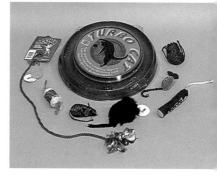

Cats love toys that stimulate the hunting instinct.

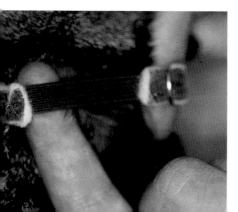

Make sure the collar you buy has an elasticated section.

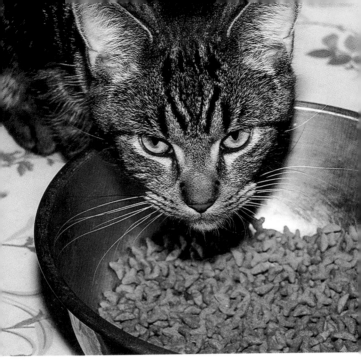

Dry food is manufactured to supply all your cat's dietary needs.

FRESH FOOD – this may be the most palatable, but you have to be very careful to ensure that your kitten gets a balanced diet. A wide variety of animal-based foods is essential, as some cats have a tendency to latch on to just one type of food such as liver or fish, and refuse to eat anything else.

CANNED FOOD – canned kitten foods are now readily available, and provide a complete, well-balanced diet for your kitten during its growth stage. Kittens should be fed with fresh food a little at a time, and unused food should be refrigerated.

DRY FOOD – this is probably the most hygienic and straightforward way to feed kittens, leaving out a complete, dry growth food that a kitten can take ad lib during the course of the day. Although some early formulations of dry cat food were thought to play a part in causing bladder problems (see feline urological syndrome page 177), this has now been corrected, and it is perfectly safe to feed just a premium quality dry cat food.

Although some kittens do not drink very much, it is important that a supply of fresh water is available at all times, especially if dry food is being fed. There is no necessity for kittens to drink milk, and cow's milk will give some of them diarrhoea due to an inability to digest lactose, the sugar found in milk. If it causes no problems, there is no harm in giving some milk – or special cat milk, with the lactose removed, can be purchased.

EARLY TRAINING
It is amazing how well kittens adapt to life in a new home, and how quickly they learn the behaviour that is expected from them.

TOILET TRAINING
A kitten is naturally clean, and will instinctively use a litter tray that is put down for it. If this proves a problem:-

- Try changing the type of litter.
- Add a little soil to the litter.
- Avoid using any strong smelling disinfectants to clean the tray.
- Ensure the tray is situated in a quiet corner where the kitten feels secure.

LIVING WITH OTHER PETS
Introducing a new kitten to other pets can be a problem. Strangely enough, it is often more difficult to get an adult cat to accept a new member of the household than a dog. It is best to give the two cats a chance to get used to each other under supervision, making sure the kitten has somewhere high up to escape if threatened. In some cases, leaving the kitten in a wire-mesh cat carrier allows them time to get to know each other without the risk of either party getting injured. With time, a new kitten usually will be accepted by other pets in a household, and will learn to live side by side with them.

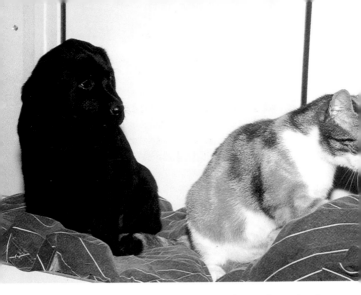

Dogs and cats can learn to live alongside each other.

Natural instincts can be curbed, but it would be very unwise to take any chance with cats and small animals.

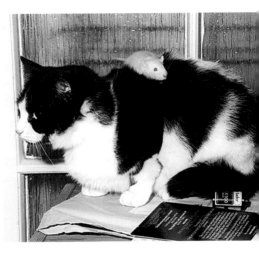

THE OUTSIDE WORLD

Once the vaccination course has been completed and sufficient time allowed for it to take full effect (one to two weeks, depending on the vaccine), you may want to start allowing your kitten access to the big outdoors. This is a cause for concern to many owners, but rarely proves to be a problem, as kittens are naturally cautious and will not generally run off and get lost.

Make sure the kitten has a collar with your name

and telephone number clearly displayed, and arrange the first outing at a time when the kitten is expecting to be fed. Most kittens will just take a few cautious steps outside and then rush in again, only gradually venturing further afield as they become more confident. Some owners are not prepared to take the risk of their cat getting run over, and make some, or all, of their garden 'cat-proof' – a task that requires some pretty impressive fencing. Alternatively, you can train your kitten to get used to being exercised on a leash. It is surprising how well cats will accept this if they are accustomed to it from an early age.

CAT FLAPS
Cat flaps are very convenient, and some will only admit cats that have been fitted with a special magnetic collar, keeping unwanted visitors out. Some kittens find it hard to get the hang of using them, and propping the door open until they become accustomed to going through it will help. Those with a transparent perspex flap may also be more readily accepted.

FIRST VISIT TO THE VET
You may want to have your kitten checked over soon after purchase to ensure all is well, and some pedigree breeders insist upon this. It is not strictly essential if all is otherwise well, but you should contact your surgery immediately for general advice on kitten care and to find out when the vaccination course should be given. This can vary, but is most commonly given at nine and twelve weeks of age. Most vets like to allow the kitten to settle in for a few days before giving a full health check and vaccination. This first visit is an excellent opportunity for you to get professional advice on any aspect of kitten care that may be causing concern.

CAR TRAVEL
If you want your cat to get used to travelling in a car, now is the time to start. Even for a long journey, it is

best not to rely on sedative drugs, as they are very unpredictable in cats. However, skullcap and valerian is a mild herbal sedative that is available in a veterinary formulation and is safe to administer to cats. Do use a spacious and well-ventilated cat carrier to keep your kitten secure. Travel sickness is much less likely if you avoid giving any food for a few hours before travelling, and get your kitten used to lots of little journeys at first.

VACCINATIONS
Vaccinations are available against feline infectious enteritis, cat flu, and feline leukaemia virus (see relevant entries in Chapter 7 for further information about these diseases). At the present time, cats are not vaccinated against rabies in the United Kingdom unless they are being exported overseas, but in the United States kittens are routinely vaccinated. All these diseases are very serious viral infections, and owners should ensure their kitten is fully vaccinated before being allowed to mix with other cats.

WORMING
Worming should be carried out regularly, particularly for roundworms, which can be passed directly to the kittens from their mother. Other parasites, such as ear mites and fleas will need to be treated if present.

IDENTIFICATION
It is now possible to permanently identify a cat with a tiny microchip that can be injected under the skin over the scruff of the neck. This gives the kitten a unique identification number that can be read with an electronic scanner. As most cat rescue centres now routinely scan cats that are brought to them, this system is a very worthwhile precaution in case your cat is lost, or if there should be any dispute over its ownership.

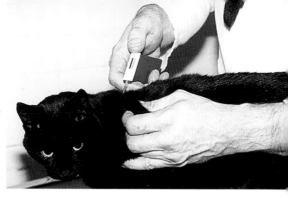

A tiny microchip can be implanted as a means of permanent identification.

INSURANCE

It is wise to take out pet health insurance while your kitten is well – it is no good waiting until a problem develops! For a relatively small monthly payment you can insure against the cost of veterinary treatment in case of accident or illness, so that all you have to pay is an excess for any course of treatment. This is not yet readily available in the United States.

ADULTHOOD

FEEDING

As the rapid growth phase slows down after six or seven months of age, the nutrient requirements of a young adult start to reduce rapidly. Feeding a diet with the same calorie content can lead to obesity, although cats are better than many other species at matching their food intake to their energy requirements.

The choice of food sources is still the same as for a kitten, but if the kitten has been fed on pre-prepared foods, then instead of feeding a food designed to support growth, a food matched to the requirements of an adult cat will be needed. This will not only have a lower calorie content, but will also have a different balance of minerals and vitamins.

HEALTH CARE

Most owners know that kittens must be vaccinated, but some forget that vaccinations need boosting annually. As well as the injection itself, this is also a vital opportunity for your cat to have an annual health examination. In this way, many impending problems can be identified and corrected before they become serious. This should automatically form part of the consultation procedure, with the vet checking your cat over to ensure that it is in good health in order to receive the vaccinations. Some practices even fill out a form at this time to emphasise that a health examination has been carried out, and to highlight any areas that need attention.

PARASITIC CONTROL

Fleas are a major problem in most temperate climates, and prevention is much better than waiting until a major infestation has established itself around the house and then trying to eradicate it. A once-a-month dose of medicine is all that is needed to keep this problem at bay, but as the most effective products are only available by veterinary prescription, you should take this opportunity to discuss flea control with your vet. (See fleas, page 181.)

Regular preventative treatment against worms, particularly roundworm and tapeworm, is also advisable, even if you do not actually see any signs of the worms themselves. If your cat is an avid hunter, then worming at least once every three months is advisable, and twice a year as a minimum. Fleas can also carry tapeworms, so any flea infestation must be cleared at the same time to prevent re-infection. Modern worming preparations will kill both roundworms and tapeworms with just one dose, without causing any undue side-effects. (See roundworm, page 231, tapeworm, page 239 and lungworm, page 208).

NEUTERING

The vast majority of pet cats are neutered before they mature sexually. Although this may sound a bit tough, there are several good reasons why this should be the case:-

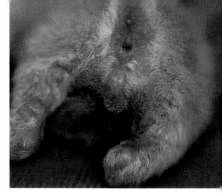

Male kitten genitalia.

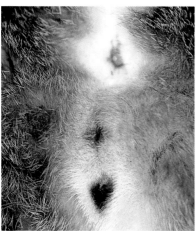

Neutered male cat.

FEMALES
•Prevents unwanted litters of kittens being born.
•Avoids the disturbing behavioural changes that occur during oestrus (see below).
•Discourages tom cats from calling, and possibly urine marking.
•Prevents certain health problems such as womb infections and breast cancer.

MALES
•Reduces the tendency to fight with other male cats over territory.
•Reduces the desire to roam and defend a large patch.
•Removes the strong male scent from their urine, and reduces the desire to urine-mark their territory.

CASTRATION
Neutering a male cat involves castration, which is surgical removal of both testicles. Naturally, this is

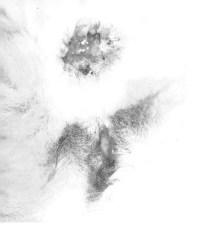

Female genitalia.

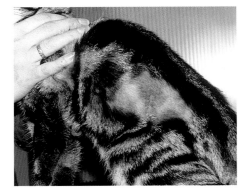

The site where a female cat has been spayed.

carried out under a short anaesthetic, needing a small incision into the scrotum (the sac that contains the testicles) that is not normally sutured afterwards, but quickly heals across on its own. The procedure is normally carried out at five to six months of age, but can be done at any time after that.

SPAYING

The surgical neutering of a female cat is normally referred to as spaying, and can be carried out at around five months of age, before she is likely to come into season. It can also be carried out in a mature female provided she is not actually in season, or in a queen that has had a litter once her milk is drying up. It can even be carried out in a pregnant female if it is essential to prevent her from having a litter, but the surgical risks are higher and the procedure is not recommended if there is any reasonable alternative.

The operation is usually carried out via a small incision in the flank, although it can be performed via a ventral midline one (an incision down the middle of the tummy). This may be desirable for aesthetic reasons with Siamese cats that are to be exhibited at cat shows after neutering, as the hair will tend to grow back darker where it has been clipped. An ovario-hysterectomy is normally carried out, which means that both ovaries and all of the womb down to the cervix is removed. It is desirable that the ovaries are removed as well as the womb, or the cat will continue to come into season despite being infertile.

ROUTINE ANAESTHESIA

Follow the directions that you are given when you make the appointment for your cat's operation. This will almost certainly involve removing any access to food after the evening meal the night before, restricting access to water a few hours before the operation, and keeping the cat in overnight.

Take your cat to the surgery in a sturdy cat carrier, clearly labelled with your name. You will probably be asked to sign a consent form, explaining that any surgical procedure carries some degree of risk, agreeing to the operation and any further procedure that should become necessary. Do not be unduly alarmed by this, as although it is a legal necessity, the risks for a routine operation such as neutering are very small indeed.

Your cat should receive a pre-anaesthetic examination, either while you are still present or after being admitted. A pre-medicant may be administered to mildly sedate the cat and assist the anaesthetic procedure. There are several different ways in which the anaesthetic itself may be administered. Most commonly it involves an intravenous injection into a vein in the forearm, possibly followed by gas administration either through a mask, or an endotracheal tube, which passes down the larynx and into the trachea. You may therefore notice that your cat has had some hair clipped from the forearm as well as around the surgical site, although some anaesthetics are administered solely by an injection into a muscle.

Your cat should be awake by the time it is returned to you, which for a routine operation such as neutering is usually later the same day. Again, follow the directions for post-operative care that you are given. Small amounts of a light diet such as fish or chicken should be fed, initially little and often, to avoid any stomach upsets. It is also important to keep your cat indoors and under observation during the recovery period. If you have been given any medication to administer, follow the directions you have been given. You may be asked to bring your cat back for a post-operative check, and if non-absorbable stitches have been used, you will need to bring your cat back to have them removed.

If you are unhappy about the way your cat is recovering from the operation, or are unsure about any directions that you have been given, do not hesitate to contact the surgery. All practices are obliged to offer a 24-hour emergency service to their clients.

BREEDING YOUR CAT

Think carefully before you take the decision to breed from your female cat. Looking after a queen and her kittens is not very difficult, but it does require a certain level of commitment and expense. It is essential that you are confident you will be able to find good homes for all the kittens, which may be relatively easy with pedigree kittens but rather more difficult with non-pedigrees. Many owners want to keep an offspring from a female cat before she is neutered, and the experience of rearing a litter is a truly fascinating one, but the decision to breed is not one that should be taken lightly.

THE SEASONAL CYCLE

If a female cat is not neutered, she is likely to come

into season before she is a year of age. The exact timing will depend upon the individual cat and also the time of year, since kittens are most commonly born during the spring and summer months. The term 'coming into season', or oestrus, means that ovaries are ready to release their eggs. It is also called 'calling', as the female may start to yowl and scream in order to try and attract a mate. Her behaviour is also likely to change – she may become over-affectionate, and pressure over her back will stimulate her to raise her rump and lift her tail to one side. Some cats even yowl and roll around on the floor so much that their owners phone their vet in a panic, thinking that their cat must be suffering from severe abdominal pain.

The cat is a reflex ovulator, which means that her ovaries only release their eggs as a response to the act of mating. This is perhaps why mating in the cat is literally a short and sharp affair. The male will grab the female by the scruff and mount her quickly. His penis has barbs along it, which cause her obvious pain when he withdraws, and stimulates her to ovulate. She is also likely to turn around and give her partner a wallop with her paw for his trouble.

With a pet cat that goes outdoors, this process will take its own course, and even in a neighbourhood where all the male cats appear to be neutered, an entire tom always seem to materialise from nowhere to mate with her. Queens will often mate with more than one tom, and it is possible for one litter to contain kittens with more than one father. If you own a pedigree queen, you will obviously have to keep her indoors when she is calling, having set up arrangements in advance for her to be taken to a stud tom for mating. Many breeders insist that a female cat is blood-tested for feline leukaemia and immunodeficiency viruses before mating.

If a female cat is not mated, she will carry on calling for about five days and then all will go quiet again. This cycle will then repeat itself about every three weeks through the breeding season until she is mated. It is possible to suppress this oestrus activity with drugs, although it is not advisable to do this to prevent the first season, or to continue with drug treatment indefinitely.

PREGNANCY

If a queen does become pregnant, all will go quiet while the foetuses develop in her womb. Sometime a female continues to call despite having been mated, or will stop calling and then start again (see infertility, page 198). The gestation period for the cat is around 63 days. In the first half of pregnancy there is little external sign that a cat is pregnant, but as the kittens develop, an owner may notice that their cat begins to 'fill out' around the abdomen, and the nipples and mammary tissue will become more prominent.

Having said this, the changes are quite subtle, and vets are quite frequently presented with cats that are 'putting on a bit of weight', when in fact they are about to give birth. It is usually possible for a veterinary surgeon to be able to palpate the abdomen of a female cat and detect if she is pregnant at three to four weeks after mating, at which time the individual foetuses can be clearly felt. After this

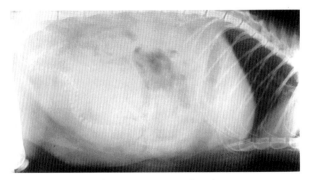

*X-ray of a pregnant cat showing
a foetus in the abdomen.*

stage, the enlarged womb becomes more difficult to feel, and an X-ray or ultrasound may be necessary to confirm whether or not a cat is pregnant.

GIVING BIRTH

Most cats do not need a great deal of assistance when they give birth, and are generally happiest if left undisturbed, with subtle observation at a distance. However, some cats are so domesticated that they insist on having their kittens in the midst of everyone.

Before the kittens are due, prepare a nesting area and encourage the queen to go to it to feed. A closed cardboard box with a hole cut into it, lined with plenty of newspaper, is generally well accepted – and it can be easily replaced when it becomes soiled. The box should be located in a warm and secluded place.

A queen may show some signs of abdominal discomfort before she goes properly into labour, and will seek out somewhere suitable before obvious straining begins. You only need interfere if the queen seems unwell and has an abnormal discharge (smelly, or dark-coloured) before labour begins, or if she strains properly for more than an hour without

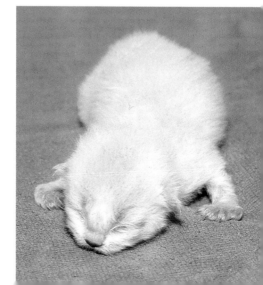

A newborn kitten.

producing any kittens. There can be a gap of several hours between kittens being born.

Even first-time mothers seem, instinctively, to know how to cope with the kittens, licking them furiously after birth to clean off the foetal fluids and stimulate breathing, then biting off the umbilical cord. A placenta (afterbirth) may be produced after each kitten, and will often be eaten by the mother. Do not worry about this, or about checking to see that the right number of afterbirths is passed. The kittens are blind and deaf, but have very good senses of smell and taste, and can usually find their way to their mother's nipple to suckle. Once a kitten establishes its place, it will return to that same nipple every time to feed.

Some kittens do not feed properly, or their mother rejects them, and it is always best to be prepared with a miniature kitten-feeder and some cat replacement milk. Ordinary cow's milk is totally unsuitable for feeding newborn kittens, but in an emergency, unsweetened condensed milk can be used. The kittens will have to be fed every two or three hours around the clock at first, and, after feeding, their abdomens must be massaged with cotton-wool to mimic the mother's licking, and to stimulate them to urinate and defaecate. The queen does not need to change her diet in the first half of pregnancy, but she will want to eat little meals more frequently as the womb enlarges and presses on the stomach. It is particularly important once she starts suckling her kittens that she has access to ample amounts of a high-energy food rich in minerals and vitamins. A food that is designed for growth is ideal for this purpose, and can also be used to feed the kittens as they wean off their mother's milk.

THE DEVELOPING KITTENS
Just as with humans, the rate of development of an infant can vary enormously from one individual to another. The approximate pattern of development is as follows:-

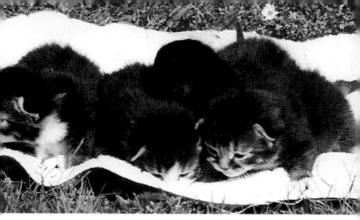
By the end of the first week, the kittens' eyes begin to open.

BIRTH
The kittens are unable to either see or hear, but they have a keen sense of smell and touch. They soon develop the ability to make enough noise to attract their mother's attention. However, they have very little reserves and will become cold and weak if they do not get their first feed within a couple of hours. Even by the end of the first day, kittens will hiss and spit at unfamiliar smells and sensations, but will grow used to humans if gently handled from an early age.

WEEK ONE
The kittens should double in weight in the first week. Their eyes are just opening, but are pale-blue at this age. They have no teeth, but they are getting better at pushing themselves around on their limbs. They spend about one-third of their time feeding, and most of the rest asleep, but will wander up to one metre (over a yard) from the nest, emitting loud cries for help if they become lost. The use of an infra-red heat lamp suspended above the nest will allow them to choose their own favourite temperature – they will pile up in a heap to keep warm and spread themselves out if they are getting overheated.

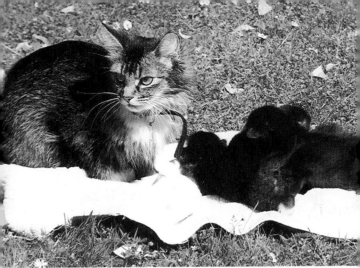

The queen will still spend most of the time with her litter.

WEEK THREE

The kittens should now have reached four times their birth-weight, and their senses of sight and hearing are well-developed. Their milk teeth are beginning to erupt. They can stand up on their legs to move around, but they are still completely dependent upon their mother for food and protection.

WEEK FIVE

The kittens can be weaned on to solid foods. Start off by teaching them to lap fluids – encouraging them to lick some milk off your finger, and then putting your finger into the dish. The kittens can then progress to small amounts of scraped meat or finely-mashed kitten food. They can now walk and run confidently, although sometimes they lose their balance and take a tumble, and they can groom themselves. Their repertoire of communication skills has to greatly extend from just cries and purrs, to enable them to express themselves to other cats and to humans.

Good socialisation is extremely important, and a kitten that is deprived of plenty of friendly human contact at this age may never develop into a fully domesticated adult. The same applies to other contacts, such as with dogs, and the kittens should

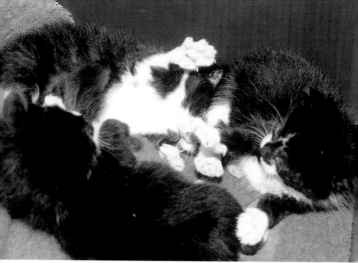
Kittens play-fighting at three weeks of age.

be carefully exposed to as wide a range of experiences as possible. The kittens are now beginning to play, which is a very important part of the learning process.

WEEK EIGHT
The kittens are now becoming fully independent. In the wild, the queen would initially bring back dead food for her kittens to eat, but, at this stage, she would start to bring it back alive for the kittens to learn to kill at this age. Once the kittens start to eat solid food their mother stops cleaning them and the time for litter training starts. This often follows quite naturally, and they will follow their mother into the litter tray that she uses, but it is important that they have somewhere available that they can dig, or they will relieve themselves anywhere.

Most queens will spend increasing amounts of time away from their kittens, and discourage them from suckling during the day. It is now time for them to go off to their new homes and to start out on the programme for kitten care outlined at the start of this chapter.

THE VETERAN CAT
A well cared-for cat can easily reach fifteen years of age, and, from time to time, they make it into their

twenties. The oldest documented cat was Puss, a tabby from Cullompton in Devon, UK, who died in 1939 at the grand old age of 36. Just as humans are now expecting to live some of their most fulfilling years after they retire, with the aid of modern veterinary science we can now usefully enhance the quality of life of many elderly cats.

FEEDING

The nutritional requirements of the elderly cat have only begun to receive close scrutiny in recent years. Unlike the dog, where there is a marked tendency to obesity in old age, some cats seem to become less efficient at absorbing their food, and actually tend to lose weight. Therefore some elderly overweight cats may need a diet mildly reduced in calories to match their reduced level of activity, whereas others may need a more concentrated source of energy.

There is certainly a need for higher levels of certain minerals and vitamins, and if a cat is showing any indication of kidney disease, protein and phosphorus levels will need to be restricted. Your veterinary surgeon will be able to recommend a diet to cater for your cat's specific needs.

Elderly cats may be less able to cope with hard foods than when they were younger, and it may be necessary to avoid dry cat foods or to soften them with some warm stock.

DENTAL PROBLEMS

Dental problems are very common in old age, due to the gradual accumulation of tartar over the years. Anaesthetics are now very safe, even for the elderly, and it should not automatically be assumed that a cat is too old to have some essential dental care carried out under anaesthesia, unless there is some specific medical condition that rules it out. Even if an elderly cat can only be given a few months of pain-free and happy life by removing badly infected teeth, most owners would consider this worthwhile.

GROOMING

An elderly cat with a sore mouth or a stiff neck may be unable to groom itself effectively, and may require extra assistance in this department.

HEALTH CARE

As well as dental disease, common problems that affect cats in old age include kidney failure, hyperthyroidism, heart failure and cancer. Arthritis is less common in the cat than in many other species, but elderly cats will gradually become stiff and less agile. All these problems are discussed in detail in Chapter 7. It is especially important that elderly cats receive a regular health examination to detect problems at an early stage.

Most vets recommend that vaccination boosters are continued throughout a cat's life. Although some viral infections are more common in young cats, diseases such as cat flu can still affect the elderly, and are more likely to lead to life-threatening complications if they do strike. Your vet may advise that your cat has a check-up more frequently than just once a year, and many practices offer 'senior pet health programmes'. This involves an in-depth health examination, usually involving a blood test, and sometimes leading to other examinations such as ECGs to measure the rhythm of the heart, and X-rays. This can be repeated every six months, or more frequently if the cat's condition warrants.

EUTHANASIA

It may seem strange to discuss euthanasia in a book about health care, but putting an elderly or sick cat to sleep is sometimes the kindest course of treatment you can offer to a dearly loved friend. The decision is never easy, but, together with your veterinary surgeon, you should be able to work out what is in your cat's best interests.

In my opinion, even cats with a terminal disease should not be denied a few weeks or months of good-quality life if their problem can be kept under control satisfactorily and without distress. But it is unfair to keep a cat going if they are getting no enjoyment from life, simply because the owner is unable to make a decision.

Cats are generally euthanised with an overdose of barbiturates, which is given intravenously into a vein in the forearm, or by injection directly into an organ such as the kidney. This type of drug is used as an anaesthetic, and in its highly concentrated form it literally sends the cat to sleep. The loss of consciousness is quickly followed by a cessation of breathing, and the heart will stop beating. Sometimes the cat may take a gasp, some muscles may tremble, and the bladder and rectum may empty. None of this is pleasant to watch, but it is purely a result of reflex activity as the oxygen supply to the muscles dies out. It is not an indication that the cat is conscious in any way. Owners are often unsure whether to stay with their cat while it is put to sleep, but those that do, are generally reassured to see how quick and painless that whole procedure is.

Most cat owners are eager to ensure that their pet is treated with respect after it has been put to sleep, and you should not be embarrassed to discuss the arrangements with the veterinary surgery. Cremation is the normal means of disposal, and the return of ashes can usually be arranged, if requested in advance.

It is not unusual to suffer from bereavement after the loss of a pet cat, particularly if you have shared a very close relationship. In some cases this can be as severe as with the loss of a close relative, and psychologists recognise that people may go through the same stages of mourning, regardless of whether the bereavement is human or animal. The important thing is to realise that this is not abnormal, or something to be ashamed of. There are organisations that offer the services of pet bereavement counsellors to help pet owners talk through their emotions.

Chapter Five

FELINE BEHAVIOUR

THE LION IN OUR HOME

The domestic cat is far closer to its wild relatives than the dog, with even the most highly-bred pedigree cats still bearing a close resemblance in size and body shape to their ancestors. One of the attractions of owning a cat is the opportunity to live

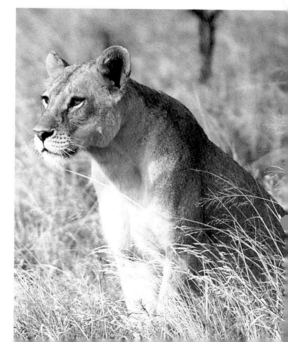

Big cats in the wild bear a strong resemblance to the domestic cat.

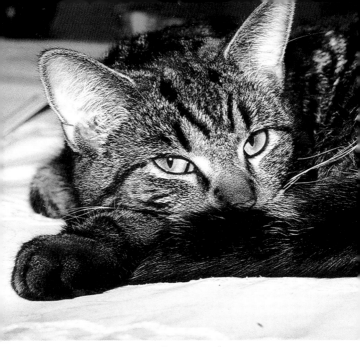

A contented cat.

side by side with a creature that is so close to nature, and would still be able to fend for itself in a feral state if necessary. The cat is basically a wild animal with a thin veneer of domestication laid over it. Feline psychologists (yes – there are quite a few!) tell us that the domestic cat has learned to live its adult life in a suspended state of kittenhood, treating its owners as it would its mother, curling up on our laps, purring when stroked, kneading us with their paws (as they would to stimulate milk flow), and dribbling in expectation of their next feed.

This usually works out fine, but we demand a lot from our domesticated cats, especially when we expect them to thrive in an indoor urban environment, or a suburban setting cramped with far more cats than they would naturally co-exist with in the wild. Sometimes the natural wild behaviour breaks through that veneer of domestication, and what may be perfectly normal behaviour for a wild cat becomes unacceptable for a domestic cat living in a human household.

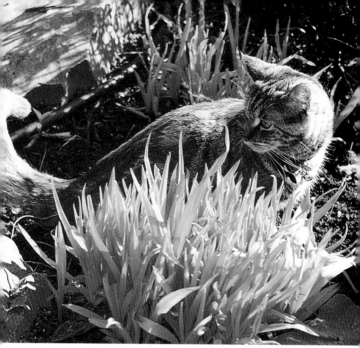

On the alert.

The mental health of a pet cat can be of just as great concern to a veterinary surgeon as its physical health, and it is not uncommon for behavioural problems to result in rehoming or even euthanasia of an otherwise healthy patient. An understanding of the normal behaviour patterns of the cat can not only give us a greater appreciation of our companions but can also help us to avoid problems occurring, and to deal with them when they do.

FELINE COMMUNICATIONS

Cats are equipped with many different means of communication, for use both with other cats and with humans. Facial communication is particularly important for humans, and we can understand a lot about our cat's mood by looking at their expressions:-

CONTENTED – the 'cat that got the cream' will be totally relaxed, with its ears forward and its eyes half-closed. A long and slow blink with both eyes is

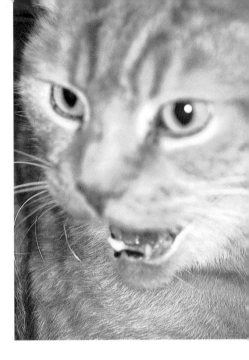

*Spitting
with
aggression.*

understood as a sign of friendship, and is expected to be reciprocated.

EXCITED – the ears prick forwards and the eyes are widely open, with dilated pupils.

FRIGHTENED – pupils again dilated, but this time the ears are flattened down against the head.

AGGRESSIVE – pupils still dilated, but ears forward and mouth open, baring a threatening array of teeth.

To cats, other means of communication are equally important. The sense of smell is particularly important to territorial and sexual behaviour. This is particularly true in the case of entire tom cats, but will apply to females and neutered cats as well. Urine and faeces are used as territory markers to inform other cats in the area of their presence, and like all carnivores, cats are equipped with anal sacs on either side of the anus that contract to secrete a strong individual scent on to the faeces.

Cats also possess scent glands in the skin above the base of the tail, on the face below each ear, and between the toes on the underside of the feet which also play an important part in determining the

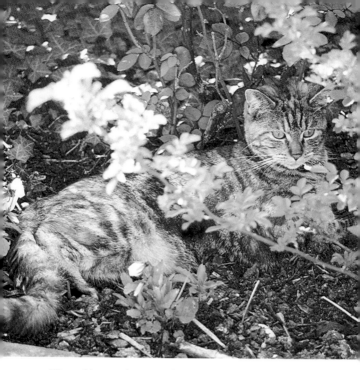

The tabby markings make good camouflage.

On the prowl.

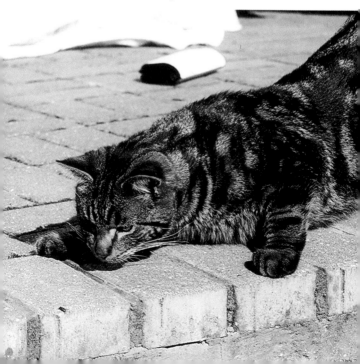

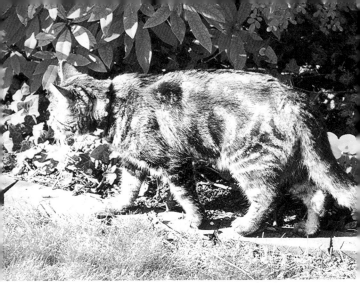

The cat retains all its hunting instincts.

The cat is naturally inquisitive.

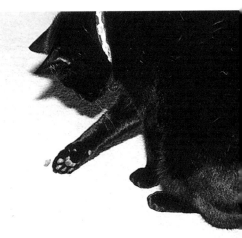

behaviour of the cat. Thus, the cat that rubs its face against its owner is not just showing affection, but also marking its owner with its own scent as a form of bonding.

Anyone that has heard a wailing tom cat at night, or the howls of a female cat that is literally 'calling' for her mate, will know that sound is also important as a means of communication. Vocal communications start with the instinctive crying of a young kitten that is calling for its mother, and the purring of its mother as she contentedly suckles her young.

Adult cats have a large repertoire of meows, chirrups, spits and growls to convey a wide range of meanings, and there is evidence to suggest that cats develop a special repertoire of sounds to communicate with their owners. We may not understand their exact meaning, but most cats seem to have developed the art of training their owners to respond to their demands very effectively!

However, feline communication does not stop there, as body language is extremely important as well. We have all seen the frightened cat that literally puts its hair on end, the tail erect and bushy, standing on tip-toe to make itself look as large and threatening as possible to frighten off its attacker. Relaxed cats will groom each other to help bonding, and the cat that is unsure about something will often give this away by a twitching or wagging of the tail.

AVOIDING TROUBLE

Many pedigree cat breeders are keen to hold on to their kittens until they have completed their vaccination course at twelve weeks of age, but there is a strong argument, from the behavioural viewpoint, for a kitten to go to its new home as soon as it is fully independent from its mother. If you want to own a cat that bonds closely with humans, it is even more important to obtain a kitten that has been handled regularly for significant periods of time, every day, from a couple of weeks of age. It has been shown that the period between two and seven weeks of age is critical in terms of accustoming the kitten to regular human contact so that they accept it as normal.

Every cat is an individual, but there is no doubt that genetic influences play an important role in determining behaviour. This applies to non-pedigree cats to some extent – tortoiseshells have a reputation for being nervy, whereas ginger cats are renowned for their placid nature. Although any generalisation can be dangerous, the genetic influence is more obvious with certain breeds that are known to have unique characteristics and to be more prone to certain behavioural disorders.

For example, very few Siamese cat owners would take issue the with statement that their cats are more vocal than most other cats – closely followed by other Oriental breeds such as the Burmese and Abyssinian. This type of cat is also more demanding of attention, and prone to indulge in destructive behaviour if ignored. The moral of this story is that if you want a quiet life – don't purchase an Oriental kitten! Whatever breed you fancy, you should take time to find out more about the nature of the breed before you take the plunge. Talking to experienced breeders at a local cat show is an ideal way to achieve this.

PRINCIPLES OF CAT TRAINING

Some people would argue that it is impossible to train a cat. It is certainly more difficult to train a cat to carry out specific tasks than a dog, but even this is possible with a lot of time and patience. Most people are not particularly interested in owning a cat that will fetch a toy when thrown, but they are keen to have a cat that is generally sociable and free from behavioural problems. In this context, we are looking more at modifying the behaviour pattern of the cat to avoid specific problems rather than training it to carry out specific tasks.

When confronted by a cat that has misbehaved, it is an understandable human reaction to show our displeasure and punish the cat, but this is rarely effective in modifying its behaviour – even if it does give us an opportunity to give vent to our feelings. If any form of rebuke is to be administered, it must be given immediately the misdemeanour occurs if it is to be any use at all. For example, it is certainly no use to come back home to discover a mess on the carpet and then scold the culprit, as the cat will not associate the punishment with the 'crime'. If the cat can be caught in the act, then with certain types of problem some form of aversion therapy may help. However, the rebuke must not be associated with the presence of the owner, or the cat will simply learn to indulge in the behaviour when the owner is not around.

For example, a cat that regularly scratches at furniture may soon learn to stop if sprayed with a jet of water from a plant-spray or a water-pistol from a distance. It sees this harmless but unpleasant punishment as an 'Act of God' that occurs whenever it scratches in the wrong place. It must be remembered that many types of anti-social behaviour, such as urine spraying, are often stress-related, and administering any form of punishment will simply raise the poor cat's stress levels and make the problem worse.

The subtle approach is usually more successful with cats, and wherever possible the owner should try and understand why the cat is indulging in the particular problem and see if steps can be taken to alleviate the cause, or direct the behaviour in such a way that it no longer causes a problem.

COMMON FELINE FOIBLES
TOILETING PROBLEMS

Messing in the wrong place indoors is the commonest problem that cat owners report to veterinary surgeons. It is important to differentiate between urine spraying as a form of territory marking, where the urine will be sprayed several inches off the ground in strategic sites, and inappropriate urination and defaecation, where the cat is simply reluctant to use its litter tray. In either instance, it is advisable for the cat to have a veterinary examination to rule out any underlying medical cause of the problem, such as cystitis.

Urine spraying is much more common in entire toms than in neuters, and their urine smells much more strongly, but even females will spray sometimes. If a cat sprays outdoors, it is usually considered acceptable, but it becomes a problem when a cat starts to spray indoors. The commonest cause is territorial insecurity, where a cat feels that its home territory is threatened, either by other cats in the household or by a cat from outside. The greater the number of cats in a household, the greater the chance of having a problem with urine spraying. Cats are likely to feel particularly stressed if they know that an outside cat is getting access to their home via a cat flap; either blocking up the flap or fitting one that is activated by a magnetic collar may ease the tension.

One interesting new treatment that is proving very useful is a product sold in the UK through veterinary surgeons under the trade name of Feliway. This is an extract of feline facial pheromone, which is the scent that cats deposit on marking posts by rubbing their faces against them. Spraying this substance around areas where a cat is urine spraying will relax them and lessen their urge to make a mark of their own. In some severe cases, a course of tranquillising drugs may be given to relax the cat and alleviate the problem.

Inappropriate urination and defaecation is more likely to be due to a reluctance by the cat to use its normal litter tray. There are several steps that can be taken to assist:-

•Make sure the cat does have easy access to a litter tray. Sometimes a cat that is used to going outdoors may feel threatened by a new cat and look for a tray inside.
•Ensure the tray is in a quiet, secluded spot, where the cat feels safe using it.
•Do not use any strong-smelling disinfectants to clean the tray – the smell may deter the cat.
•Experiment with different types of cat litter, and even try adding some soil from the garden.
•Clean out the tray regularly, as cats are very fastidious. Cleaning up soiled areas thoroughly is important, as the scent will stimulate the cat to use

the same spot again. Very effective proprietary products that completely neutralise the smell of cat urine are now available.

•If only one or two areas are being used, place a feeding bowl with food in those spots, as cats will not use their feeding sites for toileting.

SCRATCHING

As well as helping to pull off dead nails to expose the sharp ones underneath, scratching is another form of territory marking for cats, leaving not only a visual signal to other cats, but also a scent from glands situated in the skin between the toes on the underside of the feet. Scratching is a natural and necessary process, so ensure that your cat does have ready access to a suitable scratching post that is securely fixed to a wall.

If your cat is particularly keen on scratching a particular fabric or carpet, cover the scratching post with that material if possible. Pheromone products may also help with this problem. This is one type of behavioural problem that may respond well to aversion therapy, and involves lying in wait with a water-spray until you catch the cat in action. Try not to make your presence known to the cat even after you have used the spray, so avoid whoops of triumph at all costs!

AGGRESSION

There are several types of aggression recognised in cats, such as maternal aggression to protect her young, territorial aggression to defend a cat's stalking ground and predatory aggression to catch prey, or perhaps a toy that stimulates that same form of instinctive aggression. These are all considered normal, even in a pet cat, but sometimes misdirected or inappropriate aggression can become a serious behavioural problem. In some cases, a disease condition such as a brain tumour or an overactive thyroid gland may cause a change of behaviour, making a cat that is normally placid, aggressive.

Most owners reluctantly accept that there is little that can be done to prevent cats from fighting to defend their territory outdoors, but the commonest form of aggression-related problem that vets have to deal with is where fighting breaks out between cats in the same household. Although dogs and cats are classically associated as chasing and fighting with each other, they generally learn a mutual respect, and ongoing problems are rare. The situation with cats can be rather different, with one cat seeing another as a continued threat to its territory and perhaps its food source. This can persist throughout their lives, and is a particular problem when a cat that has been used to living alone suddenly has another adult introduced. It can be very difficult to predict how one cat will take to another – even two cats that have grown up together as kittens will occasionally take a dislike to each other.

There is little that can be done to alleviate the problem, other than trying to allow each cat their own space, feeding them separately and setting up different access points in and out of the house. This should allow them to establish their own territories within the house and go about their lives relatively independently, so that conflicts occur less commonly.

Aggression directed towards an owner can also be a serious problem. In some cases, such as when a cat chases after an owner's legs and pounces on them, this can be a form of misdirected predatory aggression. It can be alleviated by giving the cat more play and stimulation, and directing its hunting instincts towards more suitable targets. In other instances it can be due to fear-induced aggression, particularly in the case of a cat that has been recently introduced into a new environment. Some cats have a hereditary predisposition towards this type of behaviour, and copious contact with humans from the age of two weeks is also important to alleviate it. Only large quantities of love and kindness can gradually overcome this type of behaviour, although in severe cases a vet may be able to prescribe some tranquillising drugs to help the process along.

It is not uncommon for some cats to exhibit what is described as petting aggression, where a cat that is being stroked seems to be enjoying the experience, but then starts to become agitated and turns to bite or scratch its owner. There are many theories as to why this happens, but I have yet to hear of a truly convincing explanation. If you know your cat is prone to this type of behaviour, you will be able to detect when it starts to become agitated, at which point you should immediately cease the petting.

WOOL SUCKING AND CHEWING

It is not uncommon for young adult cats to enjoy sucking on fabric, a behaviour that presumably simulates sucking at their mother's breast and presumably provides a similar comfort to thumb-sucking in humans. This is not generally harmful in any way, but some cats, and especially Siamese, take this one step further and actually start eating chunks out of a fabric, usually wool. This does not often cause any physical harm to the cat, although the potential for causing an intestinal obstruction certainly exists, but it can be very expensive in sweaters and cardigans!

Studies are being carried out to try and understand the cause of this most unusual condition. There is some suggestion that a high-fibre diet (but not wool) may create a feeling of fullness of the stomach and reduce the desire of the cat to satiate its strange craving. Whatever the cause, it is recommended that owners of affected cats develop very tidy habits and refrain from leaving woollen items in places where the cat can get to them.

Chapter Six

FIRST AID
AND NURSING

WHAT TO DO IN AN EMERGENCY
Do not panic – it will not help you, or your cat. The
immediate priorities are:-

•Remove your cat from further danger without
putting yourself at risk.
•Take any immediate first aid steps necessary to
preserve life.
•Contact a veterinary surgeon for further advice and
assistance.

THE ABC OF FIRST AID
The three immediate priorities of first aid are -

A for Airway: Ensure that the cat is able to breathe,
especially if it is unconscious. Clear any fluid or
debris from the mouth and pull the tongue forwards,
but be very careful to avoid getting bitten.

B for Breathing: If the cat is not breathing, you can
attempt artificial respiration by compressing the
chest with your hand once every couple of seconds
to force air out of the lungs.

C for Circulation: Try to stop serious bleeding by
applying firm pressure with a bandage over the

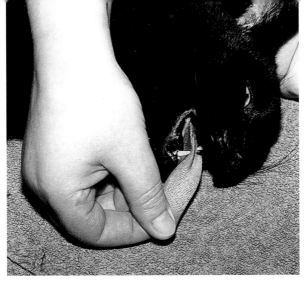

If a cat is unconscious, pull the tongue well forward to keep the airway clear.

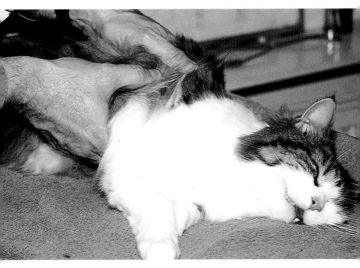

Compressing the chest manually for cardio-pulmonary resuscitation.

wound. Intravenous fluid therapy is an important part of supportive treatment that a veterinary surgeon will often decide is necessary.

Do not give anything by mouth in case the cat needs to have a general anaesthetic.

GETTING ASSISTANCE

Resist the temptation to rush straight to the nearest vet. Every veterinary surgery is obliged to offer a 24-hour emergency service, but a vet will not necessarily be on the premises at all times. If at all possible, you should telephone ahead, so a veterinary surgeon can be put on standby for your arrival. You may even be directed to another surgery that is providing emergency cover.

Keep a secure cat carrier at home in case it is required, but in an emergency a sturdy cardboard box will suffice. If the cat struggles when someone attempts to pick it up, throw a towel over it and pick it up as a bundle, placing the cat and the towel in the carrier together. Even a cat that appears unable to run far, may make a dash for freedom when frightened, so do not take any unavoidable chances. As a last resort, the cat's legs and body can be wrapped in a large towel or blanket and carried in someone's arms.

FELINE ENEMY NUMBER ONE:
THE MOTOR CAR

Once you take the decision to allow your cat to roam freely, there is little that you can do to prevent it from becoming involved in a road accident, other than keeping your fingers firmly crossed. If it is physically able, a cat will instinctively try to run off and hide after being hit, as an injured cat in the wild would not survive for long in an exposed position. External identification with a collar and name tag can be vital under these circumstances, and permanent identification with a microchip implanted under the skin (see Caring for your Cat, page 49) provides a very useful back-up.

Although a driver is legally obliged to report an accident involving a dog and many other species of domestic animal, cats are seen as 'free agents', and there is no such liability in their case. Despite this, most people feel morally obliged to stop and try to assist an injured cat. If an ownerless cat is involved

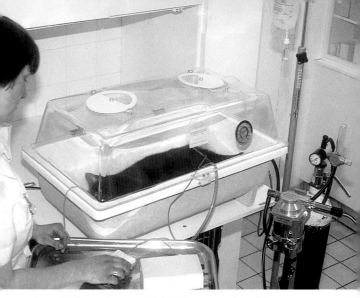

A cat in intensive care following a road accident.

in a road accident, the police (if they attend) may arrange for veterinary attention while the cat is still at the roadside. Once the cat is removed from the scene of the accident, the police are very unlikely to get involved at all. Unless you are prepared to take responsibility for the cost of the treatment yourself, it may be necessary to turn to one of the veterinary welfare organisations to assist.

A cat that has been hit by a road vehicle should always be examined by a veterinary surgeon, even if it seems unharmed externally, as there may be internal injuries that need treatment. Follow the ABC of first aid as outlined above, and make arrangements to transport the cat to the veterinary surgery without delay. If the cat is unconscious, slide it on to a towel and use that as a support to pick the cat up with the minimum of disturbance. Do not try to splint any broken bones, as you will almost certainly cause further damage as the cat struggles; and do not give anything by mouth in case an anaesthetic has to be administered.

BLEEDING
There is little that can be done in the way of first aid to assist a cat that is bleeding internally, or perhaps

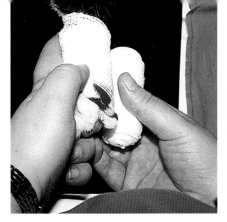

A pressure bandage can be used on a bleeding foot.

out of its mouth or nose, apart from keeping it comfortably warm and seeking immediate veterinary attention. However, it there is heavy bleeding from a wound on a limb or some other accessible spot, it may be possible to apply a pressure bandage to try and staunch the flow of blood. Ideally, you should apply a swab of sterile gauze, or some similar material, and then firmly apply a bandage over that. Within reason, do not worry about making the bandage too tight, as it will need to be removed as soon as you arrive at the veterinary surgery, and most people tend to apply pressure bandages too loosely to be of any value in stopping serious bleeding.

BURNS

These can result from heat, electrical burns or contact with corrosive chemicals. Electrocution quite commonly results from a cat chewing at electrical flex, and can cause severe burns to the mouth, or death due to cardiac arrest. It is very important to turn off the electric current at the mains before attending to the cat. Although its hairy coat provides a considerable degree of protection against both heat and chemical burns, cats will often suffer problems when they attempt to lick corrosive chemicals off their body.

The most important first aid procedure with any type of burn is to flush it very liberally under cold running water, which will cool down the damaged tissues and wash off any chemical contamination. In

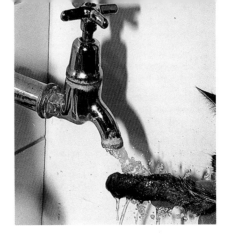

A burn should be treated with cold running water.

the case of chemical burns, you should prevent the cat from licking itself while being transported to the vet.

CHOKING

Cats occasionally get objects such as pieces of chicken bone trapped in their mouth, particularly across the roof of the mouth. Playing with a piece of cotton and then swallowing it, complete with needle, is a favourite game for many kittens. This will cause considerable discomfort, drooling and pawing at the mouth, but will not interfere with the cat's ability to breathe.

Although this requires urgent attention, an even more serious problem exists if something is obstructing the passage of air into the cat's chest. In this instance, the cat will become extremely distressed, the tongue and mucous membranes of the mouth will acquire a marked bluish tint, and collapse and death will rapidly follow. Unfortunately, reaching into the throat of a panicking cat to try and clear an obstruction is very dangerous and unlikely to be successful. If the cat is unconscious, you may be able to pull the tongue forward out of the mouth, and perhaps even grasp any foreign body visible. In a conscious cat, you could try grasping it by the thighs so that it hangs upside down between your legs, and gently swinging it back and forth a few times to try and shift the obstruction with the aid of gravity.

Failing this, you could try sharply compressing the

chest between your hands in the hope that the rapid exhalation of air forces the offending item out of the throat. Even if the obstruction has cleared, the cat should receive a veterinary examination to make sure that secondary problems are not developing due to swelling in the throat.

DROWNING

The procedure for resuscitating a cat that has stopped breathing due to drowning is very similar for choking, and again, speed is essential if there is to be any chance of success. Hanging the cat upside down and gently swinging it back and forth may be particularly effective in helping the water to drain out of the lungs. Even if the cat recovers from the original incident, there is still a significant chance of pneumonia developing as a result of the water that has been inhaled into the lungs.

FITS

It is best not to disturb a cat while it is having a fit – just make sure it is out of harm's way, preferably in a dark and quiet room, and keep it under close observation. If the fit lasts for more than about five minutes, or if the cat keeps having fits in quick succession, then urgent veterinary attention is required, otherwise the cat should be checked over once convulsions have ceased. (See fits, page 179.)

FRACTURES, DISLOCATIONS & SPRAINS

These usually occur as the result of some traumatic injury such as a road accident. A fracture is considered more serious if it is compound, which means that the skin is broken over the fracture site and infection has contaminated the break in the bone. (See fractures, page 184). The most important first aid step is to try and restrict the movement of the cat to prevent further damage. *Do not* attempt to apply a splint or bandage, as the cat will invariably struggle and you could even end up turning an uncomplicated fracture into a compound one.

Dislocations and sprains will affect a joint rather than along the length of the bone, and particularly in the former instance the cat will be very lame on the affected limb and an obvious deformity may be visible. With any of these injuries, the veterinary surgeon is likely to need to carry out an X-ray to confirm the diagnosis and establish the best form of treatment. A sprained joint may benefit from cold compresses held on it, but resist the temptation to give any anti-inflammatory drugs designed for human use, as many can be toxic to cats.

INJURIES

Minor wounds can be bathed in a solution of one teaspoonful of salt dissolved in a pint of warm water. Do not use any antiseptics or disinfectants unless you know they are harmless if ingested – for example, many antiseptics derived from coal tar are toxic to cats. Wounds very commonly become infected, especially those that result from a bite from another cat. You should seek veterinary attention if:-

* The wound is deep, gaping or open and may require stitching.
* The wound penetrates a critical area such as the chest or abdomen.
* The wound becomes inflamed, smelly, and begins to discharge.
* The cat seems unwell or refuses food.

All too commonly, youngsters decide that cats make good target practice, and it is not unusual for a puncture wound to turn out to have been caused by an airgun pellet. Sometimes they will embed themselves in muscle and cause no long term harm, but the consequences can be very serious if it penetrates a vital organ, or introduces serious infection.

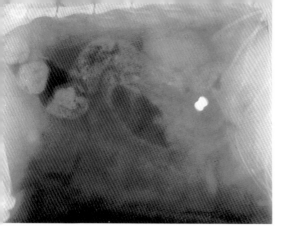

X-ray of an air-gun pellet injury.

POISONING

This subject is dealt with in Section III (see poisoning, page 221), but remember:-

• Speed is essential.
• Unless the substance is caustic, you could try to make the cat vomit while the poison is still in the stomach, by dosing the cat with a small crystal of old-fashioned washing soda, or a strong solution of salt water.
• Keep any relevant information about the nature of the poison, such as the packet in the case of pesticides.
• Contact your vet without delay.
• If your cat has contaminated its coat with a harmful substance, physically prevent it from grooming itself, preferably by wrapping its body and legs in a towel, until it has been thoroughly cleaned.

ADMINISTERING MEDICATIONS

TABLETS

If they can be given with food, crush the tablet in a small amount of strong-smelling food and offer it to the cat when it is hungry. If you have to administer the tablet whole, you should lubricate it with a little butter, and use your left hand (if you are right-handed) to grasp the head and bend it back as far as possible. The mouth will then drop open a little, and you can use one finger of the other hand to pull the lower jaw down. Quickly push the tablet right to the back of the cat's throat. You can use a special pill-holder if you do not want to risk getting bitten. It is easiest if you have someone else steadying the cat, and if necessary, you may need to wrap its legs in a towel to prevent scratching.

LIQUIDS
Bend the head back in a similar manner, and dribble the drops into the side of the mouth. Allow time for the cat to swallow, or the medicine may be accidentally inhaled.

EYE OINTMENT
Pull down the lower lid with one finger and drop the liquid or ointment into the space between the eyelid and the eye. Avoid touching the eye with the end of the dropper itself, or the surface of the dropper on to the eye. Discard any eye preparations a maximum of six weeks after opening the pack.

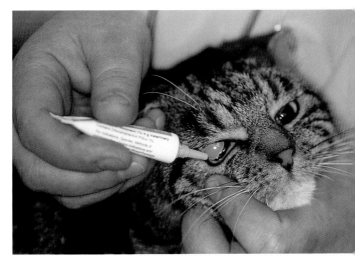

Administering eye ointment.

EAR DROPS
Ask someone to hold the cat firmly across its shoulders. If necessary, you can wrap the legs in a

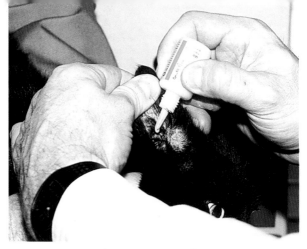

Administering ear drops.

towel to prevent scratching. Hold the ear flap firmly between the finger and thumb of one hand, and use your other hand to squeeze the bottle so that the drops drip down into the ear. Keep hold of the ear flap firmly until you have inserted all the drops. Massage the side of the ear canal to encourage the drops to run down well into the ear and to help loosen any discharge. Let go of the ear flap, wipe away any excess drops around the top of the ear canal – and wipe down the walls!

ANAESTHESIA

Many owners are naturally concerned when they discover that their pet has to have a general anaesthetic. There are many different anaesthetics drugs being used in cats, some being injected into a muscle, some intravenously, and others as a gas. The most common procedure for anaesthetising a cat for a procedure of any length would involve the intravenous administration of a rapidly acting agent to induce unconsciousness, followed by the introduction of an endotracheal tube into the airway and maintenance via that tube on gaseous anaesthetic.

In most small-animal practices the anaesthetic would be induced initially by a veterinary surgeon and then maintained by a veterinary nurse while the vet proceeds with the operation. It is normal for food

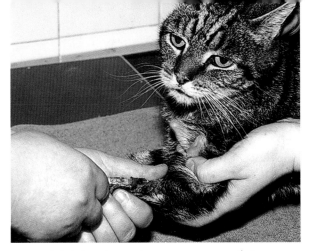

Administering an intravenous anaesthetic.

to be withheld overnight before a routine anaesthetic to reduce the risk of vomiting, so cats should be kept indoors overnight, and the practice informed if there is any chance of the cat having eaten.

Many owners are particularly concerned about the risks involved in anaesthesia if the cat is elderly. Of course, any general anaesthetic does carry some risk, even in an apparently perfectly healthy cat, but with modern anaesthetics that risk is now extremely

An endotracheal tube is put down the trachea to maintain a clear airway under anaesthetic.

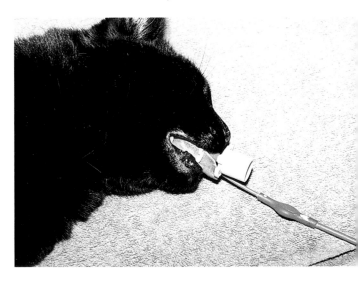

small, and even elderly cats are regularly anaesthetised for routine procedures such as preventative dental care. Some disease problems, such as cardiovascular disease, do increase the risk of complications, and the owner and the vet have to carefully weight up the pros and cons in these cases before a decision is made. Very often, the risk of not investigating or treating a problem may outweigh the anaesthetic risks involved.

POST-OPERATIVE CARE
Pay close attention to the instructions that you are given when you collect your cat after an operation. Many practices will run through the details before returning the cat, and will back up the advice with a written information sheet. Do not hesitate to telephone the surgery when you get back home if you realise there is something you have not understood. General tips include:-

•Give any prescribed medications as directed, and contact the surgery if you are unable to administer them, or if the cat seems to have any untoward reaction.
• Unless you have been told otherwise, do not give any food until the cat is fully awake, and then give just a small, easily digestible meal, such as white meat or fish with rice.
•Check any dressings or casts regularly to ensure they are not overly tight or causing excessive discomfort. Dressings will probably need to be removed after a few days, or changed regularly. Watch out for any unusual smell or discharge.
•If the wound is visible, it may well look slightly inflamed, and at first may ooze a little blood. Contact your veterinary surgeon if it becomes increasingly reddened, swollen, and hot, or if there is a significant amount of discharge or bleeding. Given the chance, a cat will always lick at a wound, but if this becomes excessive the licking may make it sore, or the cat may even pull out the stitches. It is

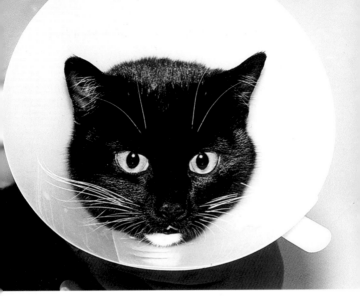

Your cat may need to be fitted with an Elizabethan collar to stop it interfering with its stitches.

sometimes necessary to fit the cat with an Elizabethan collar that fits around the neck and prevents it from getting to the wound.

• Depending upon the operation, your cat may well be off-colour while recuperating from the surgery, although after a routine or minor procedure this should not last for more than a day or two.

• Sutures are usually removed at around ten days after the operation, although in some cases they may need to be left longer. Sometimes, only absorbable sutures are used under the skin, and may not need removal.

DIETARY MANAGEMENT OF DISEASE

Cats are often very fussy about what they will eat, especially when they are unwell. A wide range of prescription diets are now available to help treat many conditions, including to help recuperation after an operation. Getting a cat to change to one of these diets may be difficult. Here are some tips that may help to change a cat to a new diet, or tempt a cat that is off its food:

• Try different formulations and brands. For

example, most prescription diets are available in either canned or dry form, and some in different varieties. Your vet may be able to supply you with a different brand if your cat refuses the first it is offered, and some cats prefer a regular change of diet.

•Change diet gradually. You may be able to fool your cat into accepting the new diet by gradually adding an increased proportion to the normal food, but attempt to feed only the prescribed food in the long run.

•Warm the food. Opening a new can excites many cats and often tempts them to eat more than an opened can taken from the fridge. Most cats prefer to have the food warmed to body temperature, making it smell more strongly. Your vet may be able to supply flavour enhancers to sprinkle on the food.

•Hand-feeding may often help to entice your cat.

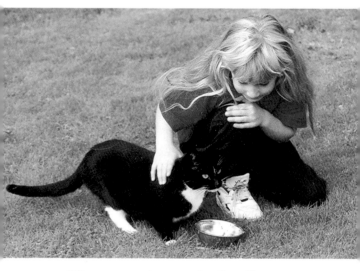

When your cat is recovering from illness, you may need to tempt its appetite.

SECTION II

SIGNS OF DISEASES AND HEALTH PROBLEMS

Section III, which follows this Section, is an alphabetical list of the health problems affecting cats , but if you are concerned about a particular clinical sign that your cat is showing, this chapter may help you to find the relevant entry in that section.

The following figures are used to indicate the degree of urgency of the particular problem, although it will also depend upon the severity of the condition:-

1. Call your veterinary surgeon immediately.

2. Call the surgery to book the next available appointment.

3. Do not panic, and arrange to see a vet when it is convenient unless the cat is otherwise unwell.

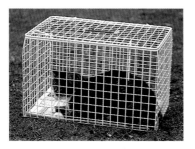

A cat should be transported to the vet in a cat carrier.

ANAL IRRITATION
Less common in cats than in dogs, the cat may be seen to be licking itself more than normal around its rear, or scooting its bottom along the ground.
DEGREE OF URGENCY 2
Possible causes: anal sacculitis (page 131), tapeworm (page 239).

BAD BREATH
Officially known as halitosis, this is most commonly due to problems within the mouth, but can be due to internal disorders.
DEGREE OF URGENCY 3
Possible causes: dental disease (page 159), gingivitis (page 187), kidney disease (page 202).

BEHAVIOURAL ABNORMALITIES
Most cat owners are very sensitive to changes in their cats normal pattern of behaviour. The cause is often

psychological, but sometimes there can be an underlying physical problem.

DEGREE OF URGENCY 3

Possible causes: brain tumours (page 139), feline infectious peritonitis (page 172), feline spongiform encephalopathy (page 176), rabies (page 228), toxoplasmosis (page 244). See also Feline Behaviour, page 77.

BLEEDING

It is very difficult for an owner to judge just how significant blood loss from their cat actually is – what one owner will describe as a 'spot of blood', another will describe as a major haemorhage. Bleeding from a major severed artery is likely to be much more serious than from a vein. Arterial blood is a bright red colour, and can sometimes be seen pumping under pressure from the damaged vessel, whereas venous blood is a darker colour and oozes from the wound. A severe loss of blood will lead to paleness of the normally pink mucous membranes, cold extremities, and extreme weakness or collapse.

DEGREE OF URGENCY 1

BREATHING, LABOURED

This will be particularly obvious after exertion, but may also be seen as 'abdominal breathing' at rest, with the cat trying to shift air into the lungs by moving its abdominal muscles in and out, rather than just the chest.

DEGREE OF URGENCY 1

Possible causes: anaphylaxis (page 132), asthma (page 135), diaphragmatic hernia (page 163), feline infectious peritonitis (page 172), haemothorax (page 190), heart disease (page 191), pleurisy (page 219), pneumothorax (page 221).

CHOKING

The larynx of the cat is very sensitive, and any obstruction or irritation of the back of the throat will result in marked signs of gagging, drooling and general distress. This can often be due to some sort of foreign body such as a fish bone or even a needle, but can be caused by irritants that have been swallowed, or insect stings. Less commonly, ulceration of the back of the throat due to infection, such as with one of the 'flu viruses, can cause similar signs. If the cat's breathing is partially obstructed, the mucous membranes and tongue may develop a marked bluish tinge due to the lack of oxygen in the blood.

DEGREE OF URGENCY 1
See First Aid and Nursing, page 90.

COLLAPSE

A cat that is normally active may suddenly go off its legs and become unable to rise. A collapsed cat will normally be lying still, although its limbs may be extended rigidly, compared to the paddling movements that will be seen if the cat is having a fit.

DEGREE OF URGENCY 1
Possible causes: anaphylaxis (page 132), heart disease (page 191), iliac thrombosis (page 198), poisoning (page 221), shock (page 235). See First Aid And Nursing (page 90) for first aid procedures.

CONSTIPATION AND STRAINING

It is important to differentiate straining to pass a motion, or constipation, with straining to pass urine, which is a much more urgent problem if a urinary blockage is present. Cats may not pass faeces for a few days after a period of anorexia.

DEGREE OF URGENCY 2
See constipation (page 153).

CONVULSIONS

See fits (page 179).

COUGHING

Acute coughing may be caused by irritation of the airways, such as by smoke or dust inhalation. Occasional coughing, especially in long haired cats, may be due to loose hairs being swallowed during grooming and causing irritation at the back of the throat. Repeated bouts of coughing may be due to a problem further down within the chest, and should not be ignored.

DEGREE OF URGENCY 2
Possible causes: asthma (page 135), bronchitis (page 140), coughing (page 154), lungworm (page 208).

DIARRHOEA

This may be difficult to spot in a cat that has ready access outdoors, and may simply show as soreness of the anus or faecal staining of the hair around its rear. Many mild cases of diarrhoea will respond to conservative treatment of a bland diet of lean white meat or fish with rice plus only water to drink. More serious diarrhoea may lead to incontinence due to the cat being unable to hold back the flow of liquid faeces, and may contain blood due to severe inflammation of the lining of the bowel. Although uncommon, this certainly must not be neglected, as death due to acute dehydration or internal bleeding can occur in less than 24 hours.

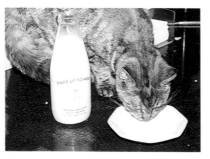

Drinking too much milk can cause diarrhoea.

DEGREE OF URGENCY 3 (unless severe or blood-stained.)
Possible causes: campylobacter (page 142), colitis (page 151), diarrhoea (page 163), giardiasis (page 186), feline infectious enteritis (page 172), intussusception (page 199), poisoning (page 221), roundworm (page 231), salmonellosis (page 233), toxoplasmosis (page 244).

EAR PROBLEMS
Signs to look out for are excessive scratching around the head, soreness of the skin around the ears, head-shaking, and an abnormal discharge or smell from the ear itself.
DEGREE OF URGENCY 2
Possible causes: ear disease (page 166).

EYE PROBLEMS
Redness of the eye, cloudiness of the normally transparent cornea, abnormal discharges or noticeable difficulty with vision, are all possible signs.

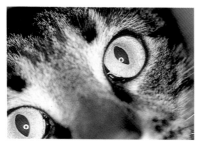

Normal eyes.

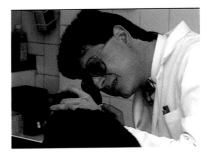

An opthalmic examination will be needed to diagnose eye problems.

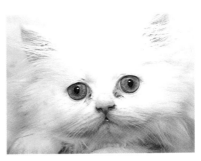

A Persian kitten with runny eyes.

Degree of urgency 2, or 1 if there is any suspicion of damage to the surface of the eye.

Possible causes: blindness (page 138), cataracts (page 145), chlamydiosis (page 148), conjunctivitis (page 151), corneal ulceration (page 153), glaucoma (page 188), Horner's syndrome (page 194), third eyelid protrusion (page 241), uveitis (page 246).

FEEDING PROBLEMS
These include:-
ANOREXIA
Not eating, or eating less than normal, which can be a sign of one of many different diseases. Remember that cats that are allowed outdoors may be getting fed elsewhere.
DEGREE OF URGENCY 2

Possible causes: gingivitis (page 187), jaundice (page 201), kidney disease (page 202), liver disease (page 206), pancreatitis (page 219), poisoning (page 221), pyometra (page 225), septicaemia (page 234), toxoplasmosis (page 244).

DEPRAVED APPETITE
Although cats generally have very finicky appetites, they will sometimes eat decidedly strange things. Although

owners often think this may be due to some deficiency in their diet, it is most commonly simply due to a behavioural quirk.
DEGREE OF URGENCY 3
See Feline Behaviour (wool sucking and chewing page 89).

HUNGER, EXCESSIVE
This may just be due to greed, but in some cases it can be caused by an underlying disease, particularly if the cat is eating a lot of food but losing weight.
DEGREE OF URGENCY 3

Possible causes: cancer (page 143), hyperadrenocortical-ism (page 194), hyperthyroidism (page 195), tapeworm (page 239), roundworm (page 231).

FEVER
It is difficult for an owner to be certain if their cat is running a temperature, but it may be suspected by the cat's behaviour or even by feeling the heat from its body. It is not advisable for an untrained person to attempt to take a cat's temperature.
DEGREE OF URGENCY 2

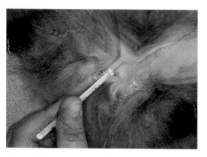

Taking the rectal temperature – this is a job for the vet.

Possible causes: abscesses (page 124), feline infectious peritonitis (page 172), feline leukaemia virus (page 174), feline panleucopaenia (page 175), keratitis (page 202), pyrexia (page 225), salmonellosis (page 233), septicaemia (page 234), toxoplasmosis (page 244).

FITS
These most commonly take the form of a 'grand mal' seizure, with a total loss of consciousness, frothing from the mouth, and paddling of the legs. Sometimes partial seizures occur, involving only part of the body, or perhaps even just a change in behaviour.

DEGREE OF URGENCY 1
Possible causes: brain tumours (page 139), poisoning (page 221).

HAIR LOSS
This is most commonly due to over-grooming that wears away the hair as it grows, rather than a failure of the hair to grow at all.
DEGREE OF URGENCY 3

Possible causes: acne (page 125), allergic dermatitis (page 126), alopecia (page 128), ringworm (page 230).

INJURIES
There are many possible causes of serious injury in cats, but unfortunately, the one that is by far the most common in built-up areas is the motor car – from glancing blows that cause just grazing and bruising, to major collisions that fracture bones, damage internal organs or even result in death. If a cat has been seen to be hit by a car but is not showing obvious signs of external injury, it should still be examined by a veterinary surgeon, as internal injuries may take time to develop. Sometimes, scuffing and shredding of the nails, caused by the cat trying to grip the asphalt of the road, will indicate that the cat has been involved in a road accident.
DEGREE OF URGENCY 1

See First Aid and Nursing, page 90.

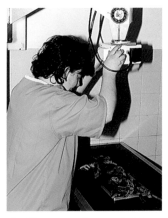

An X-ray may be needed to determine the extent of a cat's injuries.

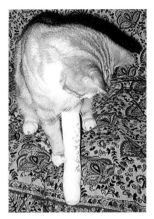

As with humans, plaster can be used for a fracture.

LAMENESS

This may be intermittent or continuous, and may affect one or more limbs. It is useful to make a note of which legs are affected, as many cats decide not to limp at all once they arrive in the veterinary consulting room!

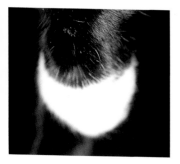

The foot has become swollen following a bite.

DEGREE OF URGENCY 2
Possible causes: arthritis (page 133), abscesses (page 124), cruciate ligament rupture (page 155), fractures (page 184), hyperparathyroidism (page 195), hypervitaminosis A (page 197), iliac thrombosis (page 198), luxating patella (page 209), osteomyelitis (page 218), spinal disease (page 237).

NAILS INGROWN

This condition is more likely to occur in elderly cats.
DEGREE OF URGENCY 2

See Caring For Your Cat, page 49.

NASAL DISCHARGE

Although a cat's nose will usually be slightly moist, there should not normally be any discharge from the nostrils. Some minor irritation may cause occasional sneezing and a clear discharge, but if the discharge persists, becomes thick and yellow, or blood-stained, veterinary treatment may well be needed. Make a note of whether the discharge appears to come from one or both nostrils. It is not normal for a cat to suffer from nose bleeds, and their occurence suggests that there may be some fairly major abnormality within the nasal passages.
DEGREE OF URGENCY 2, **or 1 if significant amount of bleeding.**
Possible causes: cat flu (page 146), chronic rhinitis (page 149).

OBESITY

It is difficult for owners to recognise when their cats are getting overweight, as the change occurs gradually. It is important to differentiate obesity from an abdominal swelling, when the musculature of the cat may be thin and wasted but the belly enlarged.

DEGREE OF URGENCY 3

See obesity, page 216.

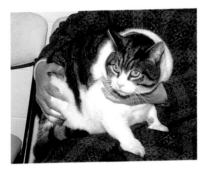

An obese cat.

PAIN

Cats often show fewer external signs of pain than a human, or even a dog, that is suffering from a similar problem. This does not mean that cats do not feel pain, although there are natural painkillers produced within the body to counteract some of its effects. However, the cat's natural reaction to pain is to hide away from danger and to be left alone. A cat that is in pain will usually resent being handled, particularly over the area that is affected. Only painkillers that have been specifically prescribed for cats should be used, as many drugs that are safe to use in other species are very toxic to cats.

DEGREE OF URGENCY 1 , if severe.

Possible causes: abscesses (page 124), arthritis (page 133), fractures (page 184), iliac thrombosis (page 198), pancreatitis (page 219).

PARALYSIS

An inability to move a part of the body, most commonly the hind limbs due to damage to the spine. If the onset of paralysis has been sudden, such as following an injury, great care must be taken in moving the cat to try and avoid causing further damage to the delicate nerve tissues.

DEGREE OF URGENCY 1
Possible causes: iliac thrombosis (page 198), spinal disease (page 237).

POISONING

If you know that your cat has been poisoned, you should contact your vet without delay, as it may be possible to administer an antidote or prevent absorption of the toxin. Never give any medicines that have not been specifically prescribed for your cat.
DEGREE OF URGENCY 1
See poisoning, page 221.

SCRATCHING

Cats tend to over-groom with their tongues rather than scratch as a response to skin irritation. The sharpness of their nails means that when they do scratch themselves, they can cause an incredible amount of damage in a very short space of time. Any topical applications are only likely to cause further irritation, and drug treatment is usually necessary to ease the irritation and treat the cause of the problem.
DEGREE OF URGENCY 2
Possible causes: ear disease (page 166), skin disease (page 236), fleas (page 181).

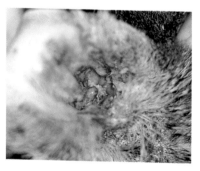

Excessive scratching can cause injury to the ear.

SKIN PROBLEMS

The most common sign of skin disease is excessive grooming resulting in areas of baldness, often combined with small scabs on the skin. Sore patches, or even just an increase in scurf can also be signs of skin disease.

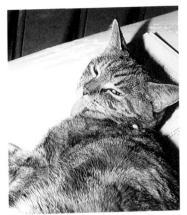

Cats are naturally fastidious and will spend long periods of time grooming themselves.

The tongue is very rough, and so if a cat is over-zealous in grooming, it can lead to skin problems.

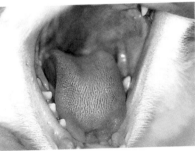

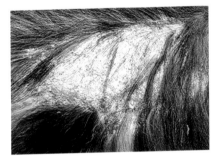

Allergic dermatitis.

DEGREE OF URGENCY *3*

Possible causes: cheyletiellosis (page 148), cowpox (page 155), feline tuberculosis (page 177), fleas (page 181), lice (page 205), ringworm (page 230), seborrhoea (page 233), skin disease (page 236), solar dermatitis (page 236).

SORE MOUTH

If a cat has a sore mouth it will usually be unwilling to eat, or will eat very gingerly. Drooling saliva, foul-smelling breath, and possibly blood coming from the mouth may be

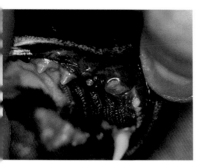

*A broken
tooth.*

noticed. The cat will sometimes paw at the mouth, and
object when a effort is made to look inside.

DEGREE OF URGENCY 2

*Possible causes: dental disease (page 159), cat flu (page
146), gingivitis (page 187).*

SNEEZING

Irritation of the sensitive lining of the nose will very often
cause a cat to sneeze. If it starts suddenly, the possibility of
a foreign body inhaled up into the nostril needs to be
considered.

DEGREE OF URGENCY 2

*Possible causes: cat flu (page 146), chronic rhinitis (page
149).*

STAGGERING

The cat normally has a highly developed sense of balance,
and any tendency to sway or stumble may indicate some
underlying problem.

DEGREE OF URGENCY 1

*Possible causes: ataxia (page 136), brain tumours (page
139), ear disease (page 166), poisoning (page 221).*

STRAINING

There are several possible causes of straining, such as
constipation, urinary disorders, or in the case of entire
females, problems with the birth process. It is important to
appreciate that a cat that is unable to pass urine must receive
immediate veterinary attention, whereas constipation is a
less urgent problem.

DEGREE OF URGENCY 1 (if unable to pass urine properly).

*Possible causes: constipation (page 153), dystocia (page
165), feline urological syndrome (page 177), intussusception (page 199).*

SWELLINGS

Cysts are discrete, non-tender masses that move freely with, or under, the skin are much less urgent than problems such as abscesses, which will be hot and tender to the touch.
DEGREE OF URGENCY 2

Possible causes: abscesses (page 124), adenomas, (page 125) anaphylaxis (page 132), eosinophilic granuloma complex (page 169), ticks (page 242).

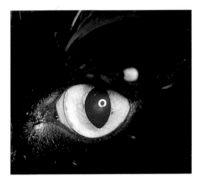

A tick above the eye.

SWOLLEN ABDOMEN (STOMACH)

It is important to distinguish simple obesity from a swelling of the abdomen due to an accumulation of fluid or a swollen organ within it. In many cases, the rest of the body will obviously be thin and wasted, despite the large abdomen, but in some cases tests such as radiography or ultrasound are necessary to determine the cause.
DEGREE OF URGENCY 2

Possible causes: ascites (page 134), constipation (page 153), feline infectious peritonitis (page 172), liver disease (page 206), obesity (page 216), pyometra (page 225), roundworm (page 231).

THIRST, EXCESSIVE

This is a common sign of illness that should not be ignored, especially in older cats. Changing a cat to a diet with a lower moisture content or a higher salt content may also cause an increase in thirst. It may be difficult to measure the water intake of a cat, particularly if they have access to outdoors, but a change in drinking pattern may be noticed. For example, a cat that does not normally drink a lot may suddenly start to drink from a tap or bowl.

DEGREE OF URGENCY 2
Possible causes: diabetes mellitus (page 161), diarrhoea (page 163), hyperadrenocorticalism (page 194), hyper-thyroidism (page 195), kidney disease (page 202), hernia (page 193), pyometra (page 225).

VAGINAL DISCHARGE

A small amount of a clear discharge may be normal in an entire female, and little vulval bleeding may be seen after mating. Any discharge that is darkly coloured or foul smelling is abnormal and should receive attention.

DEGREE OF URGENCY 2

Possible causes: abortion (page 123), infertility (page 198), pyometra (page 225).

VOICE LOSS

Whilst some cats very rarely make a noise, others (especially Siamese), keep up an almost continuous commentary. Although in these cases the peace and quiet may be appreciated, a loss of voice suggests a problem with the larynx (voice box) that needs veterinary attention.

DEGREE OF URGENCY 3
Possible causes: laryngitis (page 205).

VOMITING

It is useful to differentiate between true vomiting, where digested or partly digested food is actively thrown up from the stomach, and regurgitation, where a 'sausage' of undigested food is brought up with very little effort. Severe and repeated vomiting can be a sign of a fairly serious problem, whereas the occasional regurgitation of food is common in cats and often of no great concern.

DEGREE OF URGENCY 2 **(if severe).**
Possible causes: feline dysautonomia (page 171), intussusception (page 199), liver disease (page 206), megaoesophagus (page 210), pancreatitis (page 219), poisoning (page 221), salmonellosis (page 233), vomiting (page 247).

WEAKNESS

This can be associated with many different conditions, but is a sign that veterinary treatment should be sought without undue delay.

DEGREE OF URGENCY 2
Possible causes: anaemia (page 131), feline infectious

anaemia (page 171), hookworm (page 193), poisoning (page 221), toxoplasmosis (page 244).

WEIGHT LOSS

This may be hard to notice if it occurs gradually over a period of time; it is very common in older cats. The loss of body fat will result in a more obvious protrusion of the bony structures underlying the skin. Recording a cat's weight every few months through its life is an excellent way of picking up these changes early on.

DEGREE OF URGENCY 3

Possible causes: emaciation (page 168), cancer (page 143), hyperthyroidism (page 195), hookworm (page 193), kidney disease (page 202), liver disease (page 206), pancreatitis (page 219), tapeworm (page 239).

WORMS

Sometimes actual string-like roundworms may be vomited or passed in the faeces, or tapeworm segments may be seen stuck to the hair around the anus. However, it is possible for cats to suffer from a worm infestation without any external signs of the worms themselves.

DEGREE OF URGENCY 3

Possible causes: hookworm (page 193), lungworm (page 208), roundworm (page 231), tapeworm (page 239).

WOUNDS

Most commonly wounds in cats are caused at the result of territorial disputes with other cats, or due to injuries from prey that is being hunted. Lacerations that tear the skin open may need suturing, but puncture wounds very commonly become infected and need antibiotic treatment.

DEGREE OF URGENCY 2 **or 1 if severe.**

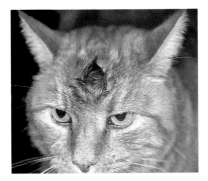

A wound sustained in a territorial fight.

Possible causes: abscesses (page 124). See First Aid and Nursing (page 90).

YELLOW GUMS AND CONJUNCTIVA

A yellowing of the body tissues due to a build-up of bile pigments in the body. It is usually most obvious in the whites of the eyes.

DEGREE OF URGENCY 2

Possible causes: jaundice (page 201), liver disease (page 206).

SECTION III

TREATMENT OF DISEASES AND HEALTH PROBLEMS A–Z

ABORTION
The loss of one or more dead foetuses before the time of normal birth.

SIGNS
Because of the furtive nature of many domestic cats, this can occur without the owner being aware it has happened. Sometimes the foetuses die and are re-absorbed back into the body without being expelled.

CAUSES
Abortion is one of the most important causes of pregnancy failure in the cat, and is most commonly due to one of a number of infectious causes such as feline leukaemia virus, chlamydia or a wide variety of different bacteria. It is thought that hormonal imbalances are not a major cause of this problem.

TREATMENT
Tests to isolate the underlying cause may identify an infection that can be treated with an appropriate antibiotic after the next mating.

ABNORMAL LABOUR
Fortunately, the birth process most frequently progresses normally and without any external assistance in cats, but it is nevertheless wise to supervise a queen in labour from a distance. See Caring for your Cat (page), for details on the normal kittening process.

SIGNS
Of course, the normal birth process involves a considerable degree of straining, but after a period of hard and continual effort, a kitten should be produced. If a queen giving birth strains for more than an hour without producing a kitten, you should seek veterinary attention without delay. A green or blood-stained discharge from the vulva before the cat goes into labour may also be a sign of a problem.

CAUSES
The two major causes of abnormal labour are either an inability of the womb to contract properly, or more

commonly, insufficient space in the birth canal for the kitten to pass through. This can be caused by a problem within the pelvis of the queen, such as narrowing caused by a previous injury to the pelvic bones, or by the size or shape of the kitten (such as a kitten that is very large, or deformed).

TREATMENT
It may be possible for a kitten that is stuck in the birth canal to be passed with veterinary assistance, but manipulation is very difficult within the relatively small confines of the feline reproductive tract, and a caesarean section is usually necessary.

ABSCESSES
A localised accumulation of pus that the body isolates off with a fibrous capsule.

SIGNS
A hot, tender swelling that often breaks open to discharge pus. These can form in any part of the body, but, in cats, they are usually found under the skin. They are one of the commonest causes of lameness in the cat, often resulting from a bite wound on a limb.

CAUSES
Abscesses are often a result of a bite from a rodent or another cat, but the bacteria that cause the problem can spread in the blood. They are one of the most common feline problems treated by vets.

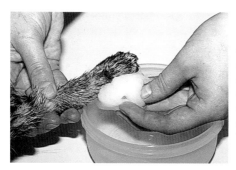

An abscess should be bathed in one tsp of salt to a pint of warm water.

TREATMENT/PREVENTION
Abscesses that are treated early with antibiotics will often subside with medical treatment alone, but once a significant quantity of pus accumulates it has to be drained off before

healing can take place. Regular bathing with a solution of one teaspoonful of table-salt in a pint of water that is as warm as the cat will comfortably tolerate, three times a day, will help to bring the abscess to a head below the skin so that it either bursts open naturally or can be lanced by a vet.

Once the abscess has burst, it is important to clean away any dried discharges and matted fur that adheres to the wound in order to keep the abscess draining for as long as possible. If it heals over too soon and more pus is trapped inside, the infection will break out again and the whole process will have to be restarted. Bathing should be continued until there is no more discharge from the wound, and the full course of prescribed antibiotics must be administered. Although both neutered male and female cats will sometimes fight, the problem is much more common in entire tom cats that aggressively try to defend a very large territory, so castration will help to prevent the problem.

ACNE
A plugging of the hair follicles around the chin area with greasy sebum, with secondary infection of the follicles with bacteria.

SIGNS
Hair loss and inflammation of the skin, sometimes with visible 'blackheads' plugging the hair follicles. It particularly affects the chin of younger cats and the tail region of tom cats, when it is known as stud tail.

CAUSES
The underlying cause is often unclear, although sometimes it can be aggravated if the cat is grooming itself excessively and rubbing its chin repeatedly against its fur.

TREATMENT
Mild cases may improve without treatment, particularly if the cause of any excessive self-grooming such as fleas is treated. A surgical scrub based on a safe antiseptic, such as chlorhexidine, can be used to regularly clean and degrease the area, but in severe cases it may be necessary to give the cat a course of antibiotic treatment.

ADENOMAS
Non-cancerous growths of glandular tissue, such as of the sebaceous glands that secrete sebum on to the skin.

SIGNS

These most commonly occur within the ear (ceruminous gland adenomas), on the eyelid, or within the thyroid gland, where they may cause hyperthyroidism to develop.

CAUSES

Not known.

TREATMENT

Adenomas are generally amenable to surgical removal as they are usually well-separated from adjacent tissues and do not tend to recur.

ALLERGIC DERMATITIS
An inflammation of the skin as a result of an allergic reaction to some triggering factor.

SIGNS

The tongue of a cat is extremely abrasive because it is armed with spines that act as a comb in the grooming process, so it only needs the cat to exert a bit more pressure

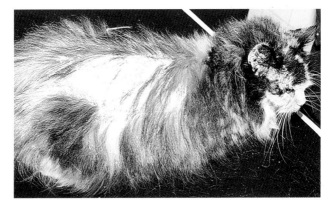

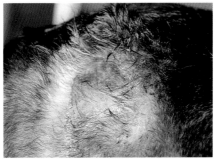

ABOVE: Severe allergic dermatitis.

LEFT: Pyoderma.

than normal while it is grooming for the hair to quickly become worn away and the skin to become raw. Therefore the signs of feline allergic skin disease may range from bald patches (where on close examination it can be seen that the hair actually is growing but is being worn away to a short stubble as it sprouts), through multiple small scabs (known as miliary dermatitis), to large sore patches that have become secondarily infected with bacteria.

CAUSES
This is by far the commonest cause of skin disease in the cat and can develop as a result of allergens that are eaten, inhaled, or more rarely, come into contact with the skin. The vast majority of cases of allergic dermatitis in cats result from an exaggerated response to flea bites, in which the cat reacts to the small amount of saliva that a flea injects when it feeds to prevent the blood from clotting. Just one flea bite can spark off an intense irritation all over its body. The importance of flea allergies as a cause of skin disease in cats was not realised for many years, and it was thought that hormonal and dietary disorders were of more significance than is now known to be the case.

Food allergies also occasionally cause skin disease, and whereas the lesions of flea allergic dermatitis are mainly concentrated around the back and tummy areas, food allergies more commonly causes irritation and subsequent self-inflicted damage around the face and neck. The allergy can develop to any foodstuff, such as a certain meat protein or a particular cereal, and the only way to diagnose the condition is to put the cat on a specially devised low-allergy diet for at least a month to see if the condition begins to improve. The infuriating tendency of cats to refuse to eat unfamiliar food, together with the difficulty of establishing exactly what the outdoor cat is eating when it is away from home, often makes this type of dietary trial very difficult.

TREATMENT
An accurate diagnosis is always the first step to effective treatment, and in cases of persistent skin disease a vet will often want to carry out tests to rule out other possible causes such as ringworm and parasitic infestations. Although laboratory tests, such as the examination of skin biopsies under the microscope may confirm an allergy as the most likely underlying cause, it will almost certainly not identify the actual triggering factor. This will often need a prolonged process of trial and error, as well as a close look at the whole

environment of the cat to try and identify it. Certainly, in any cat with chronic skin disease a determined flea eradication campaign is wise (see fleas, page 181). Since they spend so much of their life-cycle off the host, and allergic cats only need to be bitten very infrequently, fleas can often cause major skin problems and yet not be readily visible on the cat.

If the cause of the allergy cannot be identified and removed, there may be no alternative to controlling the problem rather than curing it. The long-term use of evening primrose oil, taken orally, can often do a lot to reduce the itchiness of the skin. It is produced in liquid form that is specifically designed to be added to the food of cats. Drugs such as antihistamines are sometimes of value, but most frequently long-term, low doses of corticosteroids have to be given. Fortunately, cats are pretty resistant to long-term side-effects from this type of treatment, although possible side-effects are further minimised if a short-acting corticosteroid, such as prednisolone, is used on an alternate day basis, rather than every day, or by repeated injections of a long-acting preparation.

ALOPECIA
An absence of hair from areas where it is normally present.

SIGNS
Baldness over certain areas of the body such as on the belly.

CAUSES
It can be due to the hair failing to grow, and must be distinguished from a condition such as allergic dermatitis, where the hair is trying to grow but the cat is abrading it away with its tongue as it erupts. Congenital abnormalities

Endocrine alopecia.

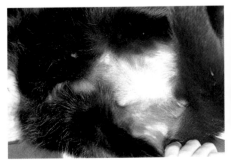

can result in alopecia, although they are rare. Hormonal imbalances have often been blamed, giving rise to what is known as feline endocrine alopecia, with hair loss over the flanks, or more commonly, on the underside of the abdomen.

TREATMENT
Alopecia often responds to treatment with thyroid hormone supplements, although affected cats do not have abnormally low blood thyroid hormone levels. It has also been speculated that male and female sex hormones may play a part in the cause, as it is more common in neutered cats and sometimes responds to sex hormone supplements. However, many veterinary dermatologists feel that although hormonal treatment may stimulate hair growth generally, the cause of alopecia in cats is not frequently caused by a hormonal imbalance.

AMPUTATION
Removal of an appendage, which in the case of the cat, may refer to a toe, a limb, the tail, or one or both ears.

SIGNS
See above.

CAUSES
Amputation of a toe may follow on from severe injury to one toe, a deep-seated infection, or a tumour. The cat is able to manage pretty well as normal with a toe missing. Amputation of an apparently normal tail may be necessary if it becomes paralysed, which may occur if the nerves to the tail become damaged by a fracture of the pelvis. Some cats cope perfectly well with a flaccid tail, and sometimes the movement does return after several months, but

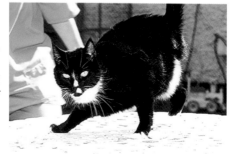

A three-legged cat can enjoy a good quality of life.

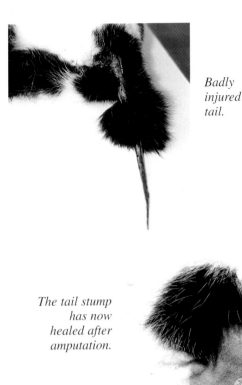

Badly injured tail.

The tail stump has now healed after amputation.

amputation is advisable if the tail becomes damaged or chronically infected. White cats sometimes develop squamous cell carcinoma, a form of skin cancer, on the tip of one or both ears as a result of long-term exposure to the sun. This type of cancer does not readily spread to other parts of the body, so can be cured surgically by amputation of the ear flaps. Amputation of a limb is not uncommon if it is severely damaged in a road accident.

TREATMENT
Surprisingly, cats generally manage extremely well, even after the loss of a limb. Many owners consider euthanasia may be a kinder alternative, but cats with three limbs generally manage to run and climb almost as normal, although it is important to ensure they do not become overweight.

ANAEMIA
A condition in which there is a reduced number of red blood cells to transport oxygen around the body.

SIGNS
Paleness of the mucous membranes in the mouth and around the eyes, combined with weakness and breathlessness due to oxygen shortage.

CAUSES
Anaemia can be caused by a failure to produce enough blood cells, their excessive breakdown, or a loss of red blood cells due to chronic bleeding, either externally or into a body cavity. Examples of each of these respectively are in bone-marrow disease due to lymphosarcoma, parasitism of the red blood cells with FIA (see feline infectious anaemia, page 171), and internal bleeding due to blood-clotting problems caused by poisoning with rat bait.

TREATMENT
A blood test may identify the cause of the problem, or it may be necessary to carry out further investigations such as X-rays and a biopsy of the bone marrow. In severe cases, it may be necessary to give a cat a blood transfusion to keep it alive while the underlying cause is being treated. In the examples quoted above, the anaemia may be improved with anticancer drugs in the case of lymphosarcoma, treatment with an appropriate antibiotic for FIA, and vitamin K injections to counteract the anti-clotting effects of rat poisons such as warfarin.

ANAL SACCULITIS
An inflammation of the anal sacs that are situated within the sphincter muscles on either side of the anus of all carnivores. They secrete a pungent-smelling fluid that is expressed on to the motions to act as a territory marker, but may also be expelled when the cat is frightened.

SIGNS
The cat will tend to scoot its behind along the ground and lick excessively at its anal area.

CAUSES
The small ducts that carry the secretion from the sacs to the skin become blocked and the impacted glands cause irritation and may become infected.

TREATMENT
A veterinary surgeon can clear the blockage by manually squeezing the glands.

ANAPHYLAXIS
An acute allergic reaction to some foreign substance that causes cells within the body to suddenly release a chemical known as histamine into the blood.

SIGNS
The signs that result from an anaphylactic reaction relate to oedema, the accumulation of excessive amounts of fluid in certain parts of the body. This may be most obvious under the skin of the head and limbs, causing a marked 'puffiness' of the ears, eyes and feet. If this oedema occurs in the lungs or around the larynx, it can interfere with breathing and cause death by asphyxiation. Sometimes the sudden release of histamine can simply cause death due to shock.

CAUSES
This reaction occurs most commonly to substances that are eaten, or to drugs that are injected or taken orally. It occurs almost immediately after exposure, although, as with any other form of allergy, sensitisation has to take place to the foreign substance at the first exposure and a reaction will only occur on subsequent contact. Occasionally an anaphylactic reaction is seen after vaccination or an antibiotic injection, although in the former case this is increasingly uncommon, as vaccines are much purer than they used to be, so less likely to stimulate an untoward response.

TREATMENT
A severe anaphylactic reaction can be life-threatening, and should always receive prompt veterinary treatment. A human antihistamine such as chlorpheniramine, which can be purchased without a prescription from a pharmacy, can be kept to hand in case of emergency, especially if a cat is known to be sensitive. However, like all proprietary medications, it should only be given on the advice of your vet. If a cat has shown a previous mild reaction to vaccination, it may be possible to suppress this by giving some antihistamine treatment before the vaccine is administered, but the owner and cat should stay close to the surgery for a while afterwards so that prompt assistance is close to hand if needed.

ARTHRITIS
An inflammation of the joints.

SIGNS

The primary sign of arthritis is pain and stiffness in the inflamed joints, which may lead to lameness if limb joints are involved. If the joints of the spine are affected, the cat may show an unwillingness to climb and to groom itself. The joints themselves may feel hot and thickened, especially if infection is present. A veterinary surgeon may be able to detect crepitus, a grating sensation that can be felt as the joint is moved. Radiographs are often needed to confirm the diagnosis.

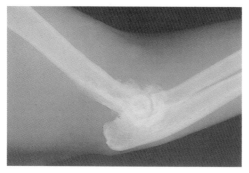

X-ray showing arthritis in the elbow joint.

CAUSES

Both humans and dogs are very prone to degenerative osteoarthritis, but this is much less common in the cat. It results in damage to the cartilage and the formation of new bone around the joint. It can occur as an ageing change, but more commonly in the cat, it is a result of some previous injury to the joint such as damage to the ligaments that support it. Given their tendency to get involved in fights, cats are more prone to suffer from infective arthritis, an inflammation of the joint caused by an infection that may be due to penetration of one particular joint. This may spread to one or more joints in the body in the blood stream from an infective source such as an abscess. Occasionally, arthritis can be caused by a disorder of the immune system, where the body's immune system attacks the joint tissue, as in rheumatoid arthritis.

TREATMENT

Ideally, any course of treatment for arthritis should attempt to correct the underlying cause of the problem, although this is not always possible. Infection must be treated with an appropriate antibiotic if it is thought to be caused by bacteria, and any structural joint problem such as torn ligaments may need surgical repair.

Long-term medical treatment may be needed to control chronic arthritis, and in overweight cats a determined effort to reduce the calorie intake will help to reduce wear and tear on the joints. Great care must be taken in the use of proprietary remedies, as many of the anti-inflammatory agents that are safe to use in other species are toxic to the cat. Even natural remedies can sometimes be dangerous. For example, cod-liver oil is often taken by humans to help with arthritis, but it contains large quantities of vitamin A that can actually cause bony inflammation in cats (see hypervitaminosis A, page 197).

There are some non-steroidal anti-inflammatory drugs (NSAIDs) that can be safely used for the long-term alleviation of pain in cats suffering from arthritis, and sometimes low doses of corticosteroid drugs such as prednisolone are used, particularly in cases of immune-mediated arthritis.

ASCITES

The accumulation of excessive amounts of fluid within the abdomen.

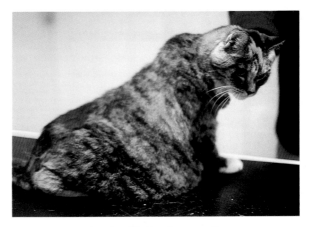

A cat suffering from ascites.

SIGNS

Distension of the abdomen, often accompanied by lethargy and a gradual loss of condition.

CAUSES

Common causes include feline infectious peritonitis, liver disease, and abdominal tumours.

TREATMENT

Ascites suggests the presence of some serious underlying disorder, and further diagnostic tests are usually required to try and establish the cause. This may include analysis of the fluid, blood tests, and radiography of the abdomen after some fluid has been drained off. Unfortunately, the physical drainage of fluid will only provide temporary relief as it will quickly re-form unless the underlying cause is treated.

ASTHMA

Respiratory inflammation as a result of an allergic reaction to inhaled substances.

SIGNS

The main sign of feline asthma is usually a cough, but it may take the form of breathing that is more laboured than normal. The diagnosis of asthma involves a blood test as well as a thorough physical examination, which will help to distinguish it from feline bronchitis – another common cause of a chronic cough.

It may be necessary to examine the cat under anaesthesia to radiograph the chest and perhaps even take a 'tracheal wash' by introducing a small amount of saline solution into the airways and sucking it back out to examine the cells microscopically.

CAUSES

Humans often develop asthma as a result of a reaction to the inhalation of substances such as pollen and housedust-mite droppings, and sometimes cats react in a similar way, although skin reactions are much more common (see allergic dermatitis, page 126). The allergens that trigger off asthma in humans can cause the same problem in cats, and pollen allergies will occur seasonally in the summer months, whereas a housedust-mite reaction will be more common in the winter when most cats spend more time indoors. Other much rarer but possible causes of asthma in cats include allergic reactions to cigarette smoke and even to human dander – the dead skin cells that all mammals shed constantly.

TREATMENT
As with any allergy, the ideal treatment is to isolate the cause of the reaction and remove it, but this is easier said than done. Improved ventilation and acaricidal sprays can help with mite allergies, and keeping the cat indoors when the pollen count is at its highest may help with cats that react in the summer. The long-term use of anti-inflammatory drugs such as prednisolone, a corticosteroid, or antihistamines, are often the only way to control the problem.

ATAXIA
An incoordination of movement due to a problem with the sense of balance.

SIGNS
It may be associated with other signs such as circling, a head tilt and nystagmus – a side-to-side flickering of the eye.

CAUSES
The most common of the many possible causes of ataxia is infection of the inner ear (see ear disease, page 166), which usually develops as a result of an untreated infection in the external ear canal that ruptures the eardrum and enters the deeper structures. However, it can sometimes originate from a throat infection that travels up the eustachian tube that connects the back of the throat to the middle ear.

Cats may also suffer from idiopathic feline vestibular syndrome, which is often described as a 'stroke', as the signs mimic the same condition in humans, with a sudden loss of balance and co-ordination that gradually improves with time. The cause of the syndrome is not known, but it is thought to be due to a clogging up of the arteries with fatty deposits – as in humans. Brain tumours may cause gradual ataxia to develop, especially in older cats.

TREATMENT
If infection is the cause, then antibiotics will help, often combined with anti-inflammatory drugs, which may even give a reasonable remission from clinical signs in slow-growing brain tumours. Cats suffering from idiopathic feline vestibule syndrome generally make good improvement if given time and careful nursing.

ATOPY
An allergic reaction to inhaled substances such as pollen, or housedust mite faeces.

SIGNS
It can affect primarily the skin or the respiratory system, causing either allergic dermatitis (page 126) or asthma (page 135), or occasionally a combination of both, and is sometimes seasonal.

CAUSES
It is not known why some animals develop this sensitivity, but it is suspected that there is a hereditary tendency to the condition. It is much less common in cats than in dogs or humans.

TREATMENT
Unfortunately, it is not often possible to avoid exposure to the allergens that trigger off the problem, although good ventilation and acaricidal sprays may help reduce the number of housedust-mites – and help any human asthma sufferers as well. Long-term dietary supplementation with evening primrose oil may help, but often it is necessary to use antihistamine or corticosteroid drugs to control the signs.

AUJESZKY'S DISEASE
This is also known as pseudo-rabies. It is a viral disease primarily of pigs that can sometimes affect cats.

SIGNS
Restlessness, severe skin irritation, leading to coma and death within 48 hours of onset.

CAUSES
It is still common in pigs in most of Europe and America, so the disease will continue to be seen in those areas where cats come into contact with infected pigs.

TREATMENT
There is no treatment or vaccine to prevent the problem, but, fortunately, an eradication programme for this disease in pigs has proved very successful.

BENIGN TUMOUR
A general term given to a non-cancerous type of growth.
See adenomas, page 125.

BLADDER DISEASE
See feline urological syndrome, page 177.

BLINDNESS
Loss of vision in one or both eyes.

SIGNS
A dilated pupil that is unresponsive to light and obvious behavioural changes indicating a difficulty with seeing objects in the cat's path.

CAUSES
Often due to physical injury to the eye itself, such as during a road accident, but sometimes due to damage to the part of the brain responsible for recognising images. If the normally clear cornea at the front of the eye, or the lens behind the pupil, become opaque, then blindness will result. The retina at the back of the eye is responsible for detecting the visual image, and in the Abyssinian, the Persian and the Siamese breeds, hereditary degeneration of the retina leading to blindness has been reported.

Feeding a cat on a vegetarian diet is likely to lead to a deficiency of the amino acid taurine, which can also cause damage to the retina. Sudden blindness can result if the retina becomes detached from the back of the eye, and this is most commonly due to a rise in blood pressure caused by an underlying problem such as kidney disease (see nephritis, page 213) or an overactive thyroid (see hyperthyroidism, page 195). Unfortunately, it is very difficult to measure blood pressure in a cat, so sudden blindness in one or both eyes may occur before it is realised that the primary problem exists.

TREATMENT
There are many cats that have lost the sight of one eye, yet live a completely normal life, climbing trees and catching

wildlife as normal. Loss of vision in both eyes is obviously much more problematical for the cat and the owner. If it occurs gradually, the cat often learns to adapt to the problem and will rely more on other senses such as smell and touch (via its whiskers), and will gradually learn its way about the house. Many cats can cope with blindness if they live in a protected environment – provided the furniture is not moved around too often! If a cat suddenly becomes blind it is likely to be very distressed and disorientated, and euthanasia is usually considered the kindest option.

BRAIN TUMOURS
A growth within the brain that may, or may not, be cancerous.

SIGNS
This can cause signs such as ataxia (see page 136), abnormal vision, abnormal behaviour, and possibly convulsions.

CAUSES
The tumours may develop either as primary lesions within the brain itself, or as secondary tumours that have spread from elsewhere in the body, although this is not common in the cat. Primary tumours of the brain are not always cancerous, but because the soft tissue of the brain is enclosed within the bony case of the skull, as the tumour expands, pressure builds up and brain damage results.

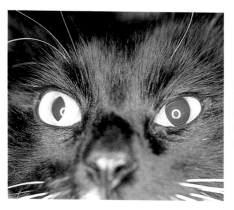

Unequal pupil size: This may indicate a brain tumour.

TREATMENT
Medical treatment with corticosteroids, and anticonvulsants if necessary, may alleviate the signs and give the cat an

extra lease of life, as some tumours only grow slowly. As most tumours involve the soft tissue of the brain rather than the skull bones, they do not generally show up on an X-ray. However, magnetic resonance imaging (MRI) scanners are now coming into use to accurately locate them, and a few cases have been successfully cured surgically.

BRONCHITIS
An inflammation of the bronchi, which are the tubes that branch out from the trachea (windpipe) into the lungs.

SIGNS
A chronic cough that has to be distinguished from that caused by irritation of the airways in feline asthma.

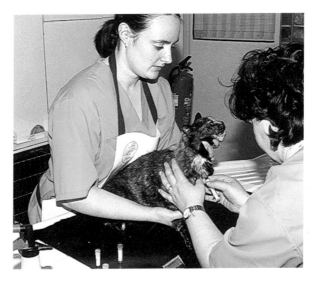

A blood sample may need to be taken for accurate diagnosis.

CAUSES
Most commonly due to a chronic bacterial infection.

TREATMENT
Tests such as blood analysis, an X-ray of the chest, and in some cases, an examination of washings taken from within

the airways with a catheter can confirm the diagnosis, and the latter will allow a bacterial culture to try and identify the cause of the infection. Bronchitis will usually respond well to a fairly prolonged course of antibiotics, but does have a tendency to recur.

BURNS
Heat damage to the skin.

SIGNS
Inflammation and sometimes blistering of the skin.

CAUSES
The hairy coat of the cat generally protects it well against the effect of burns. White cats generally have little hair on their ears, and so are prone to sunburn on the ear tips, and as with humans, repeated sunburn can lead to cancerous changes in the skin. Another part of the cat that is not protected by hair is the pads of the feet, and cats (especially kittens) will sometimes jump up on to a hot surface and blister the skin under their feet.

Electrical burns can also be a hazard, particularly when cats chew at live wire, causing very nasty burns within the mouth. Chemical burns can also cause ulceration within the mouth, because the cat will lick off any contaminants that get on to its coat.

TREATMENT
The first step with any thermal burn is to cool down the affected area with copious amounts of cold water for several minutes. Chemical contaminants should be washed off the coat, or the cat should be prevented from licking itself, until veterinary assistance is obtained. In the case of electrical burns, first ensure that the power supply is switched off.

Sunburn can be prevented by keeping the cat out of the sun during the summer, or protecting the ear tips with a non-toxic titanium dioxide-based suntan cream (although the cat will tend to groom this off quite quickly).

Severe burns will result in blistering of the skin, which then has to be protected while it heals. If a large area of skin is involved, skin grafts may be needed. Ulceration of the tongue may well stop the cat from eating, and although the tongue heals quickly, the cat may need to be fed via a tube directly into its stomach in the meantime.

CALICIVIRUS
The feline calicivirus is a small virus particle that is only infectious to members of the cat family.

SIGNS
This virus is one of the major causes of cat flu (see page 146). Some strains of the virus can cause the cat to go off-colour, run a temperature and show signs of joint and muscle pain without any evidence of respiratory disease. Some cats show these signs after they have been vaccinated.

CAUSES
The infection is spread from cat to cat, generally by sneezing.

TREATMENT
The most common strains are included in the flu vaccines. Cases of lameness due to the virus get better within a few days without any treatment. There are no drugs that will specifically kill the virus.

CAMPYLOBACTER
A bacterium found in the cat's intestine.

SIGNS
This bacterium can cause diarrhoea in cats, although cats can act as a carrier without showing any signs of ill-health.

CAUSES
It is of some significance because the organism is a common cause of stomach upsets in humans, especially young children. It is thought that cats do not often act as a source of infection for people, but the possibility should be kept in mind if a cat is diagnosed as suffering from the condition. It can be confirmed by culturing a swab taken from the faeces, although the sample has to be transported to the laboratory without delay.

TREATMENT
Oral fluid therapy, and, in some cases, antibiotics. Routine

hygienic precautions to prevent cross-infection to people or other animals.

CANCER

Cancer is not one condition, but a term that is used to describe any form of malignant growth. A cancerous growth may have a tendency to invade surrounding tissues and recur locally if removed, or it may be likely to spread to other parts of the body very early in its development, forming secondary tumours in sites around the body, called metastases.

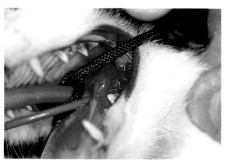

An oral tumour.

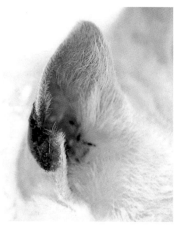

Squamous cell carcinoma on the ear.

SIGNS
Whereas benign tumours generally only grow slowly, do not invade the tissues around them and do not spread to other parts of the body, malignant tumours invade and destroy the tissue in which they originate and are likely to spread both to adjacent tissues and to other parts of the body, causing a general loss of condition as well as signs relating

specifically to the organs affected. The division between benign and malignant growths is not always clear-cut, with some cancers being highly malignant, and others being much less likely to invade other tissues in the body. They will generally cause a swelling of the body tissue involved, and may also cause problems due to the production of other substances such as fluid that builds up within the chest or abdomen, or hormones in the case of tumours of the glandular tissue.

CAUSES
The cause of many cancers in unknown, but some can be triggered by repeated irritation from a carcinogen, or cancer-promoting agent. For example, in female cats it is known that long-term treatment with drugs that mimic the effect of the female hormone progesterone can increase the chances of breast tumours developing, and repeated sunburn of the ear of white cats can result in a type of tumour known as a squamous cell carcinoma developing on the ear tips. There is some evidence to suggest that a particular type of growth, known as a fibrosarcoma, can develop at the site of vaccination in the scruff of the neck, although it is estimated that only one in 10,000 vaccinated cats develops this problem.

By far the most common cause of cancer in cats is infection with feline leukaemia virus (see page 174), which can cause a cancer of the white blood cells known as lymphosarcoma to develop. This may manifest itself within the blood but, more frequently, it causes tumours to develop around the body, and particularly within the lymph nodes, such as those found adjacent to the intestines. In young cats, lymphosarcoma most commonly develops in the thymus gland.

TREATMENT
The diagnosis of cancer is not always straightforward. An obvious mass on the body can be removed and sent off to a laboratory for analysis, or if complete removal is not feasible, a biopsy specimen can be taken. Sometimes, sufficient material for diagnosis can be obtained by a needle biopsy, a minor procedure where a needle is pushed into the mass and used to suck back some cells. A cat with a malignancy will usually be eating more than normal, yet losing weight and body condition. Specific signs of illness will relate to the organs affected by the growth – for example, a cat with tumours in its kidneys will eventually

show the signs normally associated with kidney failure, such as bad breath, inappetance and excessive thirst.

Cancer is no longer necessarily a death sentence for a cat, but early diagnosis is vital to improve the chances of successful treatment, so it is essential that the cat receives prompt veterinary attention. The ideal form of treatment for any cancerous growth is complete surgical removal, and this is often possible, although the cancer may already have spread without this being obvious at the time of surgery. Surgery may be very straightforward if the tumour is situated superficially in an area with plenty of loose skin, but may require major reconstruction if it is in a more inaccessible site such as within the bone of the jaw.

Some tumours may not lend themselves to surgery, and especially in the case of lymphosarcoma, very effective chemotherapy regimes have been devised to control the problem. Anti-cancer drugs are not generally used in as high doses as they are in humans, and the aim of treatment is usually to control the cancer and give the cat an extra lease of life, without most of the troublesome side-effects that can be associated with more aggressive chemotherapy. The most advanced form of cancer treatment for animals is radiotherapy, sometimes coupled with surgery. This is only available in a few referral centres around the country, and has to be administered on a regular basis under deep sedation or general anaesthesia to prevent the animal from moving around during the procedure.

Even with the most up-to-date treatments, there are still some cancers that are not amenable to treatment, and in these cases the veterinary surgeon has to work together with the owner to ensure the cat is kept comfortable and contented until the time that euthanasia becomes the kindest option.

CARDIOMYOPATHY
The commonest form of heart disease in the cat (see heart disease page 191).

CATARACTS
An opacity of the lens within the eye.

SIGNS
Initially a cloudiness of the lens, which may eventually lead to blindness. As a cat ages, it is normal for the lens to lose it crystal clearness and develop some cloudiness, but this

only develops slowly and does not usually lead to total loss of sight.

CAUSES
This condition can be congenital, or it may be the result of an injury or disease, or secondary to sugar diabetes (see diabetes mellitus page 161).

TREATMENT
Provided that the light-sensitive retina at the back of the eye is functioning normally, sight can be restored by an operation to remove the lens, and, just as with humans, this is often carried out using specialised laser equipment.

CAT FLU
An upper respiratory infection specific to cats.

SIGNS
The two most important causes are Feline Herpesvirus (FHV) and Feline Calicivirus (FCV), and each will tend to cause somewhat different signs. They are highly contagious and spread in the mucous secretions by coughing and sneezing. FHV generally causes the most severe disease, with runny eyes, nose, and excessive salivation. The cat often feels very unwell indeed, will run a temperature, and refuse to eat or drink. Sometimes the virus attacks the surface of the eye, causing nasty ulcers that can even lead to loss of sight.

FCV often causes milder signs, most commonly with ulcers around the mouth and on the tongue, although it can sometimes cause pneumonia to develop. From time to time, the virus can also cause lameness in one or more joints,

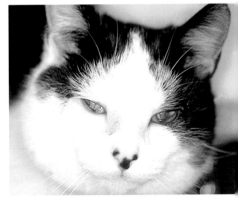

A victim of cat flu.

especially in kittens, without any of the cat flu signs that might be expected.

CAUSES
As well as FHV and FCV, there are several other agents that can cause flu-like signs, but cats cannot catch influenza or colds from humans.

TREATMENT
Topical antiviral drops are sometimes helpful for eye ulcers caused by FHV, but generally all that can be given is antibiotics to control secondary bacterial infection, and supportive treatment with oral or intravenous fluids to prevent dehydration. Careful nursing is particularly important, cleaning away discharges from the nose and eyes regularly and gently tempting the cat to eat mushy, strong-smelling foods that have been warmed to blood heat.

Cats that have been infected with the cat flu viruses may remain carriers for a long time – for life in the case of FHV, and for several months with FCV. A cat severely affected by FHV, especially early in life, may develop a persistent conjunctivitis or rhinitis (runny nose) for the rest of its life, that often tends to get worse when the cat is stressed, such as when it enters a cattery or gives birth to kittens, so it is readily passed on to other cats at this time.

A vaccine to control the cat flu viruses became available in the 1970s. Most of the vaccines are administered in injectable form, but one of the flu virus vaccines is designed to be given as drops into the nose. Although this vaccine gives a very good protection and takes effect very rapidly, it is not widely used nowadays. This is partly due to the difficulty of trying to administer the vaccine to an uncooperative cat, and partly because there does seem to be a higher incidence of post-vaccination side-effects, such as sneezing, afterwards.

Generally, the injectable flu vaccinations work well, but they will not be effective if a cat is vaccinated when it is already a carrier of FHV. Additionally, there are several strains of FCV, and although the vaccines protect against the most common strains, sometimes, just as with the human flu vaccine, a strain of virus comes along that is not included in the vaccine.

CAT SCRATCH FEVER
A disease of humans that can be contracted from cat bites or scratches.

SIGNS
Cats can carry the organism without showing any ill-effects at all, and in humans the disease is usually very mild. Some swelling around the wound may be seen, followed by enlargement of the nearby lymph glands which may take several months to return to normal. In rare cases, where the person's immune system is compromised by disease problems, such as human immunodeficiency virus (HIV) infection or the administration of immunosuppressive drugs, the organism can spread to other parts of the body such as the brain and the bone marrow and cause severe illness.

CAUSES
The condition is thought to be caused by a bacterium with the catchy name of Bartonella henselae.

TREATMENT
If any signs of illness develop after being bitten or scratched by a cat, obtain medical advice without delay.

CHEYLETIELLOSIS
A parasitic disease of the cat's skin, sometimes referred to as 'walking dandruff'.

SIGNS
Irritation and scurf, especially along the back. Sometimes the first sign is an itchy skin rash that can develop on the owner.

CAUSES
This disease is caused by mites that live on the surface of the skin that can just about be seen with the naked eye as small, white moving specks. It can also affect dogs and rabbits.

TREATMENT
A vet can prescribe a parasiticidal preparation to kill the mites. The problem on the owner's skin will clear once the pets are treated.

CHLAMYDIOSIS
Infection with an organism that mainly causes chronic conjunctivitis.

SIGNS
In cats, it primarily causes conjunctivitis (see page 151), although this can be combined with relatively mild flu-like signs.

CAUSES
Chlamydia psittaci belongs to a group of organisms that were originally thought to be viruses due to their small size, but are now considered to be a very unusual type of bacteria.

TREATMENT
It can be treated with the tetracycline antibiotics, although several weeks of treatment are needed to clear it completely. A vaccine against Chlamydia is available at the present time, although it is often only given in a cattery situation where cats are known to be at particular risk. Different strains of Chlamydia can affect many species, including humans, and as the cat agent has been associated with a few cases of conjunctivitis in humans, it is advisable to take normal hygienic precautions to prevent cross-infection such as hand-washing after petting or treating an infected cat.

CHRONIC RHINITIS

Also known as 'chronic snuffles', this is a long-standing inflammation of the lining of the nose, and is often combined with a chronic sinusitis – an inflammation of the chambers in the bones of the skull that connect to the nasal cavity.

SIGNS
Recurrent bouts, or continual sneezing and nasal discharge that is usually thick and yellow, and sometimes even streaked with blood. Since cats are very reluctant to eat food that they are unable to smell properly, the condition may cause the cat to stop eating, although, in many cases, the cat is perfectly well despite the discharge.

CAUSES
The most common cause of this condition is recurrent bacterial infection that follows on from damage to the lining of the nose caused by a severe bout of cat flu (see page 146), particularly with feline viral rhinotracheitis virus (FVR). Sometimes fungal infections can occur within the nose, or foreign bodies can enter the nostril. Tumours within the

nose itself are not very common, but they can occasionally spread there from other parts of the body.

A rather unusual condition that affects cats is nasopharyngeal polyps. These are benign (non-cancerous) growths that usually develop deep within the ear as a result of long-standing ear infections, and then grow down the eustachian canal that connects the middle ear to the back of the throat. Radiographs and a thorough examination under general anaesthetic is usually necessary to differentiate the causes of chronic sinusitis, and sometimes it is necessary to have a sample of discharge or even a small biopsy specimen examined by a laboratory.

TREATMENT
Unless a specific cause, such as a foreign body or polyp, can be identified and removed, the treatment of this condition is often frustrating. Prolonged courses of antibiotic treatment, often combined with drugs to loosen the mucus, usually result in a marked improvement, but there is a high likelihood of the discharge recurring once treatment is stopped. Taking the cat regularly into a steamy room, such as the bathroom at bath-time, may also help to clear the nasal passages. However, repeated courses of antibiotic treatment are often needed to keep the problem under control.

CLEFT PALATE
A failure of the left and right palates on the roof of the mouth to fuse together during development in the womb.

SIGNS
Affected kittens will fail to suckle normally, and will tend to inhale milk up into their nose which may be seen to bubble out of the nostrils. Nasal infections and even pneumonia often develop, and the kitten will fail to thrive.

CAUSES
This is a congenital condition (present at birth), that may be hereditary (passed from one generation to the next) in some, but not all, cases.

TREATMENT
Although surgical reconstruction is possible in mildly affected kittens, it is not usually considered desirable in

such tiny animals, and euthanasia is normally the best option.

COLITIS
An inflammation of the colon, or large intestine.

SIGNS
It tends to cause the cat to pass frequent, soft stools, often together with some fresh blood and mucus.

CAUSES
The irritation of the colon can be sparked off by bacterial infection, parasites, or, most commonly, a sensitivity to something in the diet. The problem often goes undiagnosed in the cat because of their furtive toilet habits, and may only be spotted if the cat has an accident indoors.

TREATMENT
A change to a bland diet such as boiled chicken or white fish and rice will often alleviate the problem, although more severe cases may require long term anti-inflammatory drug control.

CONJUNCTIVITIS
An inflammation of the conjunctiva, a membrane that lines the surface of the eye and the inner lining of the eyelids to form what is known as the conjunctival sac.

SIGNS
Reddening of the conjunctivae, sometimes with chemosis, a marked fluid accumulation under the conjunctiva causing it to bulge outwards. There is usually a sticky yellow discharge, and often signs of itching and rubbing.

CAUSES
This is a very common condition in the cat, and can be due to many different causes. Minor injuries, and physical irritation of the eye with substances such as pollen or dust can inflame the conjunctiva. This can then lead to a secondary infection with bacteria that are normally found in the conjunctival sac, but take advantage of the weakened defence mechanisms to multiply out of control.
  Infections can be passed from cat to cat, and conjunctivitis is frequently seen as part of a more generalised problem such as cat flu. Chlamydia primarily causes conjunctival

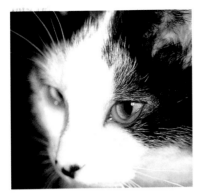

Conjunctivitis.

Chemosis.

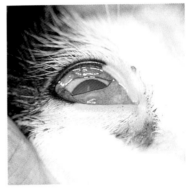

signs and is described under its own heading (see page 148). Deformities of the lids or ingrown eyelashes can irritate the surface of the eye and cause conjunctivitis, and in longhair cats with flattened faces, the hairs of the nose can rub the eye and irritate it.

TREATMENT
The administration of aqueous (water-based) ophthalmic eye-drops or ointment. Aqueous drops may be easier to apply, but they are washed out of the eye very quickly, and ointments can be administered less frequently. Applying an eye preparation is a two-person task with all but the most placid of cats, and some may even need to have their limbs wrapped into a towel for restraint.

The lower eyelid should be pulled gently downwards with one finger, and the other hand used to drop the preparation on to the surface of the eye. Care should be taken to ensure the dropper does not come into contact with the eye itself. Follow the storage and expiry directions on the medication closely, as an out-of-date drug preparation can actually introduce infection into the eye rather than cure it! No ophthalmic preparation should be used more than six weeks after opening.

CONSTIPATION
Difficulty in passing motions.

SIGNS
Owners will often notice their cat straining to defaecate, or an absence of motions in the litter tray. Care must be taken in male cats to distinguish this from a urinary obstruction (see feline urological syndrome page 177). Large quantities of faeces may build up, distending the abdomen and sometimes causing inappetance and vomiting.

CAUSES
It is common in the cat, and is often aggravated by swallowing excessive amounts of hair and indigestible foreign material (such as feathers!). It can be caused by a physical obstruction constricting the rectum, such as a tumour, or following a fractured pelvis from a road accident.

TREATMENT
Mild cases may respond to treatment with a laxative such as liquid paraffin, which passes through the intestines to lubricate and soften the faeces, but care should be taken to avoid repeated dosing with mineral oil-based laxatives as this can lead to a deficiency of fat-soluble vitamins such as Vitamin A. More severe cases may require the administration of an enema under anaesthesia to clear the obstruction. Faecal softening agents such as wheat bran (a tablespoonful a day), or similar proprietary agents, are suitable for long-term preventative treatment, although frequent grooming will also help to reduce the amount of hair that is swallowed.

CONVULSIONS
See fits, page 179.

CORNEAL ULCERATION
Damage to the transparent cornea at the front of the eye.

SIGNS
This can be a very serious problem, as, if the ulceration is

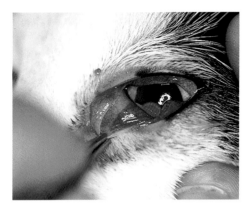

Corneal ulcer (dyed green with fluoroscein).

deep, it may penetrate the cornea completely and cause blindness. The eye will look painful and inflamed, and the cornea may appear cloudy. A green dye called fluoroscein can be used by a vet to highlight ulcerated areas.

CAUSES
Ulceration can result from physical injury or by infection that penetrates deeply.

TREATMENT
In mild cases, medical treatment with antibiotics will be sufficient to keep infection at bay while the ulcer heals naturally, but sometimes surgery is needed. This may simply involve suturing the eyelids together over the eye to act as a natural bandage, or transplanting a piece of conjunctiva over the defect. Complete corneal ruptures have to be repaired very quickly if there is to be any hope of saving vision. Soft contact lenses are now being used, in some cases, to protect the cornea while it heals.

CORONAVIRUS INFECTION
See feline infectious peritonitis (page 172).

COUGHING

SIGNS
Relatively uncommon in cats, although when it does occur, it tends to be an irritating, chronic problem.

CAUSES
Unlike many other animals, coughing in cats does not tend to be associated with lung problems such as pleurisy,

pneumonia and fluid accumulation due to heart disease, where the primary sign tends to be dyspnoea, or laboured breathing, but is far more likely to be due to irritation of the upper airways. The three main conditions that cause coughing in cats are chronic bronchitis, asthma and lungworm infestation.

TREATMENT
See under bronchitis (page 140), asthma (page 135), and lungworm (page 208).

COWPOX
A virus used by Edward Jenner in 1796 to provide the first-ever vaccination against another closely related virus, smallpox.

SIGNS
The cat may show signs of non-specific illness for a few days before the characteristic small, reddened nodules appear on the skin, especially around the head and ears.

CAUSES
Although, as its name suggests, it does infect cattle, causing lesions on the teats, it is most commonly found in wild rodents and is contracted by cats when they get bitten by one. It has been reported as infecting cats in most European countries, and is most common in rural areas.

TREATMENT
There is no specific treatment for the condition, and it usually clears up if left alone unless the immune system of the cat is suppressed by some other illness or treatment. It is possible for this virus to be transmitted from an infected cat to a human, so strict hygienic precautions should be taken in handling any infected cases.

CRUCIATE LIGAMENT RUPTURE
As any footballer will know, the two cruciate ligaments are responsible for maintaining the stability of the knee joint.

SIGNS
Because cats are generally much lighter than dogs, the injury occurs less commonly, but when it does it causes severe lameness.

CAUSES
The cruciate ligaments can easily be torn if the knee joint is twisted awkwardly.

TREATMENT
Strict exercise restriction for up to five months will almost always allow the other ligaments that surround the joint to strengthen sufficiently to compensate for the damage, but a return to normal mobility will occur more rapidly if an operation is carried out to stabilise the joint.

CYSTITIS
See feline urological syndrome, page 177.

DANDRUFF

A term used to describe a dry and scurfy coat. See cheyletiellosis (page 148) and seborrhoea (page 233).

DEAFNESS

A loss of hearing.

SIGNS

It can be difficult to assess whether a cat is deaf or not, particularly since most cats have a tendency to ignore their owners a lot of the time! It is possible to assess a cat's hearing by measuring the electrical activity of the brain in response to electronically generated sounds, but this requires light anaesthesia and is not often carried out.

CAUSES

Some cats are congenitally deaf, and this is particularly common among cats with a white coat and blue eyes, although not all such cats are born unable to hear. Damage to the ear, especially the deeper structures behind the ear drum, or to the part of the brain responsible for hearing may result in deafness, and in older cats the hearing often becomes gradually less acute.

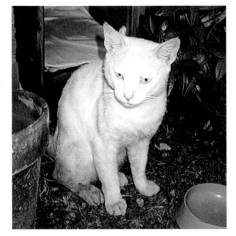

Deafness may occur in blue-eyed white cats.

TREATMENT
Cats that are unable to hear are obviously more likely to be involved in a road accident and should be kept under close control, but apart from that, deaf cats seem to manage pretty well. There is rarely any treatment for the condition.

DEHYDRATION
An excessive loss of water from the body.

SIGNS
The eyes will look dull and sometimes sunken. The cat will be depressed, and if a fold of skin is picked up along the back of the cat, between finger and thumb, it will tend to remain tented when released.

The pinch test shows that this cat is dehydrated.

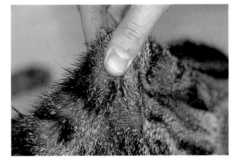

CAUSES
It can either be due to insufficient intake, such as when a cat refuses to eat or drink because it is unwell, or to excessive loss, which will occur with severe vomiting and/or diarrhoea. Cats are very good at conserving their fluid losses, and it is not unusual for a healthy cat to obtain almost all the water it needs from the fluid that is present in the food that it eats, as well as that which is produced within the body when it is burned up to produce energy. Dehydration is a potentially serious condition, since circulatory collapse can result.

TREATMENT
If a cat is able and willing to drink, oral rehydration powders are available in sachet form to be made up with water, containing the ideal concentration of glucose and minerals to aid its absorption from the intestines. They are ideal for cats suffering from diarrhoea, and even if a cat has been vomiting, they will often stay down if given little and

often. In cases of severe dehydration, or where it has not been possible to persuade the cat to drink, intravenous fluid therapy is sometimes necessary. A catheter is placed into a vein and the solution administered via a saline drip.

DENTAL DISEASE

Just like humans, cats sometimes need dental treatment if their teeth develop problems due to injury, tartar accumulation or inflamed gums.

SIGNS
Discoloration of the teeth, reddening of the gums, bad breath. Eventually loosening and loss of teeth will cause a painful mouth and difficulty with eating.

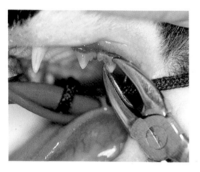

Tartar being removed.

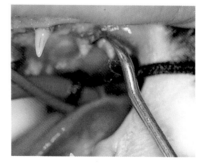

Dental scaler.

CAUSES
Pretty much any cat that lives into middle age or later will begin to develop dental problems, although some cats seem to have problems at a much earlier age than others. Of course, injury to the teeth can break the hard crown, but the commonest problem results from a gradual accumulation of

a hard, brown mineral deposit called calculus on the teeth. This pushes back and inflames the gums to cause gingivitis, which can be seen as redness and sometimes bleeding.

As the gums recede, soft dental plaque, which is an accumulation of food and bacteria, gathers on the teeth and within the pockets that form at the gum margin. This infection then spreads to the ligament that surrounds the root of the tooth and holds it into its bony socket, a condition known as periodontitis that eventually results in loss of the tooth.

Cats can also suffer from a peculiar condition where the enamel covering one or more teeth is eaten away to expose the sensitive pulp cavity underneath. Although the effect is similar to human dental caries, it is actually caused by the cats own dental-manufacturing cells reversing their normal function and reabsorbing the enamel instead of laying it down. It is not known why this occurs.

TREATMENT

It used to be accepted that as a cat got older it would gradually lose its teeth, but the process is often a painful one, and we are now aware that a lot can be done to prevent it. Diet plays a part in the condition, and food that exercises the teeth such as dry cat food or some raw gristly meat will certainly help. Some cat owners are even able to brush their cat's teeth, and special dental kits are available.

Once a significant amount of calculus accumulates and the gums become inflamed, it is unlikely that a change of diet or tooth-brushing will remove the cause of the problem, and ultrasonic descaling under a light anaesthetic becomes necessary. Teeth with badly infected roots will have to be extracted, but in milder cases it is sometimes possible to treat the gums. Teeth with a significant degree of enamel decay usually have to be extracted.

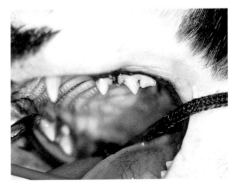

Teeth after descaling.

DIABETES MELLITUS

An increased blood-sugar level due to a problem with the action of the hormone insulin within the body (also known as sugar diabetes).

SIGNS

Affected cats develop a ravenous appetite and thirst, yet generally lose weight. As the disease progresses, toxic substances called ketones build up in the body, which can often be detected on the breath since they have a very pungent and characteristic smell, resembling nail-polish remover. In the later stages of the disease, cats become very depressed, refuse to eat, and will eventually collapse and die. Blindness may result from damage to the blood vessels at the back of the eye.

As the level of glucose builds up in the blood, it spills over into the urine, and so the condition can easily be diagnosed by the presence of glucose and ketones in the urine, or increased blood glucose levels on a blood test. Great care has to be taken not to arrive at a false diagnosis, as blood-sugar levels can rise very quickly in the cat as a result of stress, such as if the cat is restrained to collect a blood sample. Therefore, the best way to collect a urine sample for testing is at home – a procedure that will have to be repeated regularly to monitor the treatment if the diagnosis is confirmed.

In order to collect the sample, purchase some aquarium gravel of a similar coarseness to cat litter from an aquarist shop. Rinse the litter tray and the gravel thoroughly under running water and confine the cat in a room with the litter tray filled with aquarium gravel. If the cat is not used to using a tray, it may be best to get it used to ordinary litter first. Pour off the urine from the bottom of the tray into a suitable container. Your vet should be able to supply you with a bottle – if you use a food jar, ensure there are not traces of sugar left in it, or it could result in a false reading.

CAUSES

The pancreas is a small organ that lies between the stomach and the small intestine. It has two very important jobs to do: producing enzymes to digest food, and producing insulin to regulate blood-sugar levels. Insulin increases the rate at which glucose is taken up by the cells from the blood and stored as fat, thereby lowering the level in the blood. Diabetes is usually due to a shortage in production of insulin by the pancreas, although it can also be due to a resistance by the cells in the body to its effect.

Exactly why this should happen is not known, but it is not an uncommon condition in the older cat and obese cats (who are more likely to develop the condition). Longterm treatment with certain drugs, and particularly some of the hormone tablets such as megoestrol acetate that are sometimes used to treat skin problems, can play a part in inducing diabetes. It can also be caused by persistently high levels of cortisone in the blood, either due to treatment with corticosteroids, or due to an underlying case of hyper-adrenocorticalism (page 194).

TREATMENT

Once the diagnosis is confirmed, the only effective treatment is regular injections of insulin, since oral drugs are thought to have untoward longterm side-effects in cats. A change in diet may help to control blood-sugar levels, but this is rarely sufficient alone. Most owners are very concerned at the thought of having to inject their cat daily, but as the needle used is extremely fine and since the skin over the scruff of the neck is not very sensitive, cats rarely seem to object. Once treatment has started, it is essential that the cat has a very regular lifestyle and continues to receive the injections without fail throughout its life.

Initially the urine has to be collected and tested daily, although this can be reduced once the cat is on a steady dose of insulin. The cat is initially started on a low dose that is gradually increased until there is only a trace of glucose in the urine – some vets prefer to do this initially with the cat hospitalised, although the insulin requirement may alter somewhat when the cat settles into a different routine on its return home.

By keeping the insulin at a dose where there is still just a trace of glucose in the urine, the vet can be reasonably sure that the blood-glucose levels are not dropping too low. A low blood-sugar level can be as dangerous as one that is too high, resulting in weakness, coma and even death if left untreated. The owner of any diabetic cat should have some glucose powder to hand, as this can be diluted in water and is very rapidly absorbed if given by mouth to a diabetic cat that is showing these signs.

Weight control is a very important part of the treatment, to the extent that some cats with diabetes that start on insulin and then lose weight are able to cease the injections, although this must only be done under close veterinary supervision. Many owners are able to overcome the initial problems in adjusting to owning a diabetic cat, and many cats carry on with treatment and live an otherwise normal life for several years after the initial diagnosis has been made.

DIAPHRAGMATIC HERNIA
A tear that develops in the diaphragm, a muscular sheet dividing the chest cavity from the thorax.

SIGNS
Breathing difficulties.

CAUSES
If a cat receives a sharp blow to its chest, such as from a road accident, a tear may develop in the diaphragm. The condition can be diagnosed on an X-ray of the chest, but sometimes it is not discovered until some time after it occurs. Occasionally, cats may be born with this condition.

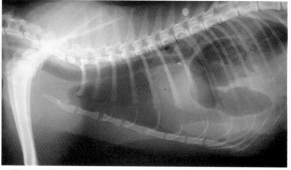

X-ray of a diaphragmatic hernia. Dark gas shadows present in the stomach can be seen within the chest.

TREATMENT
An operation to repair the tear is necessary, because otherwise an organ, such as part of the liver or the stomach, can pass up into the chest and cause severe problems. Great care has to be taken to time the operation so that the cat has recovered from the shock of the accident itself.

DIARRHOEA
The passing of soft or liquid faeces.

SIGNS
Increased frequency and urgency of passing loose motions. The cat may be obviously unwell and not eating, but not

necessarily, and in the latter instance it can be quite difficult to spot the problem in a cat that defaecates outdoors. Faecal staining of the coat under the anus may be noticed, especially in long-haired cats, and the cat will usually drink more fluids to make up for that lost in the faeces. In severe cases, blood may be seen in the motions (dysentery), and in chronic cases the cat will often lose weight.

CAUSES
This may be associated with inflammation of the large bowel (see colitis, page 151), but is more commonly due to a disease of the small intestine. Causes include the ingestion of toxins in the food, bacterial or viral infection, or parasites such as a single-celled parasite called giardia (see giardiasis, page 186). Sometimes a sudden change in diet can cause problems, as can feeding excessive amounts of milk, due to an inability to digest lactose, the sugar found in milk.

More longterm problems can be associated with lymphatic tumours that invade the lining of the intestine and interfere with the absorption of food, or other generalised diseases such as liver or kidney failure. Cats are also prone to a chronic inflammation of the bowel, called inflammatory bowel disease, that can be due to a sensitivity to some substance in the diet, but often develops with no known cause.

TREATMENT
Many cases of diarrhoea will settle down with conservative treatment, feeding a bland diet such as chicken and rice and withdrawing milk completely from the diet. Kaolin suspension can also be safely administered to slow down the passage of food through the bowel, and stool consistency regulators can be added to the food to absorb excess fluid. Veterinary advice should be sought for any case that persists for more than three or four days, or if the motions are very watery or bloody.

Again, many cases of diarrhoea seen by vets will respond to symptomatic treatment, but sometimes further tests are necessary to try and identify the cause of the problem. The faeces can be cultured for bacteria such as campylobacter or salmonella, that are known to be associated with food poisoning in both cats and humans, and checked under the microscope for parasites. In extreme cases, it may be necessary to take an intestinal biopsy, surgically removing a small piece of intestine for examination by a pathologist. Specific treatments such as antibiotics or in the case of inflammatory bowel disease, anti-inflammatory drugs may be given.

DYSTOCIA
A difficulty with the birth process.

SIGNS
Fortunately, in most cases the birth process of the cat is completely normal and can take place without any interference from the owner. However, a cat in labour should be observed from a distance to ensure all is proceeding normally, and veterinary assistance sought if a cat is straining hard and continually for more than an hour without success.

CAUSES
It can be due to a problem with the kitten, such as a deformity or being excessively large, or with the mother, such as a narrowing of the birth canal following on from a pelvic fracture earlier in life. In some cases, the uterus simply fails to contract properly.

TREATMENT
Because the birth canal is relatively so narrow in the cat, it is very unusual for a vet to be able to remove a kitten that has become lodged without carrying out a caesarean section.

EAR DISEASE

This can either affect the outer ear, which comprises the ear flap (or pinna) and the external ear canal which transmits sound down to the ear drum, or the inner parts of the ear beyond the ear drum. This includes the three tiny bones that conduct the sound in the middle ear and the deeper organs of the ear responsible for the senses of hearing and of balance.

SIGNS
Inflammation of the external ear canal is called otitis externa, and will tend to cause head shaking, scratching, pain, redness, discharge and an unpleasant smell from the ear. If infection crosses the ear drum, or travels up the eustachian tube that connects the middle ear to the throat, deafness – with or without a loss of balance – may result (see ataxia, page 136).

CAUSES
A common cause of otitis externa in cats is ear mites – very small, eight-legged parasites that commonly live in the external ear canal. They cause irritation of the lining of the canal, which stimulates the ear canal to produce large amounts of dark wax, which they then feed upon. The mites are frequently passed from a mother to her kittens, and seem to trouble some cats a lot more than others. Otitis externa can also develop as the result of bacterial infections, yeasts, polyps within the ear canal, foreign bodies, or as part of a more generalised skin infection.

In 1868 Charles Darwin recognised that white cats with blue eyes were often deaf. A few cats with this colouring are not deaf, and indeed, some white cats with different eye colours are deaf. Cats may also be born deaf if their mother has been exposed to certain viral infections or toxic substances during pregnancy. Several antibiotics can cause deafness if administered to cats, and this may remain even if treatment is stopped. It is also not uncommon for elderly cats to become hard of hearing due to a degeneration in the organ of hearing (see deafness, page 157).

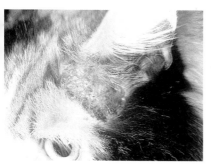

Skin trauma due to ear infection.

TREATMENT

The ear flap is frequently torn during sparring matches between cats, and although minor nicks will heal if left alone, longer ones will require stitching to help them to heal and to staunch the bleeding. White cats are prone to skin cancer due to repeated exposure to sunlight on the bald, non-pigmented skin at the tips of their ears (see cancer, page 143), and sometimes a blood vessel may burst within the ear flap itself, causing it to swell up to form an aural haematoma. If left untreated, this will contract down and leave a distorted 'cauliflower ear', which may then tend to close up the external ear canal and cause longterm ear problems. Vets can operate to drain off the blood and stitch the layers of the ear flap together to try and prevent the problem from recurring.

Ear mites lay eggs that are very resistant to treatment, so it is important that all the cats in a household are treated with appropriate drops for three weeks to clear them completely. If an owner is unable to effectively administer

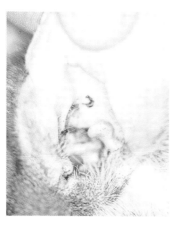

A build-up of wax due to ear mites.

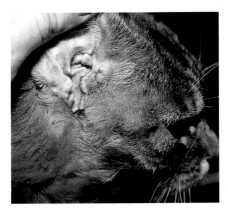

*Post-operative:
aural resection.*

drops, it is possible to give a couple of injections of a drug known as ivermectin to kill off the mites. As this product is only licensed in the UK for use as a cattle wormer (and for heartworm in dogs in the US), and has not been properly tested for use in cats, it is generally only used as a last resort. Drug treatment, usually topically with appropriate drops or ointment, will often cure bacterial infections. In the case of growths within the ear canal or very deep-seated infection, it may be necessary to carry out an operation to open up the side of the ear canal (an aural resection), or sometimes even to remove it completely.

Otitis media and otitis interna, affecting the middle and inner ear, are much more difficult to treat, as drops administered into the external ear canal are unlikely to penetrate deeply enough. Sometimes a course of treatment with antibiotic tablets will do the trick, but in severe cases it may be necessary to carry out a bulla osteotomy. This is an operation where the surgeon breaks into the bony chamber at the base of the skull that surrounds the middle ear to clean out accumulated pus and allow drainage of the infection.

ECZEMA

This is a very non-specific term that can be used to describe a chronic inflammation of the skin. It is not generally used by veterinary surgeons because it can be applied to many different skin conditions, but the most common cause is an allergic reaction to flea bites (see allergic dermatitis page, and skin disease page).

EMACIATION

A loss in body condition, also known as cachexia.

SIGNS
Loss of weight, prominence of the bony skeleton due to a
diminished covering of fat and muscle, often accompanied
by lethargy and physical weakness.

CAUSES
A cat may not be taking in food, it may not be absorbing it
properly, or it may be burning it up too fast within the body.
Cats often refuse to eat, particularly if they are running a
temperature or are unable to smell their food, such as with
cat flu. Providing that the cat is taking fluids, failing to eat
only becomes life-threatening if it persists for a
considerable length of time – weeks rather than days.

TREATMENT
As always, treating the underlying disease is the key to
solving the problem, but the section of this book on nursing
care contains information on tempting a cat to eat when it is
off its food. Failing to absorb food properly may be due to
a digestive problem (see diarrhoea, page 163) or intestinal
parasites (see roundworm, page 231 and tapeworm, page
239), whereas burning up food too quickly is often
associated with malignant tumours (see cancer, page 143) or
an overproduction of thyroid hormone (see hyperthyroidism
page 195).

EOSINOPHILIC GRANULOMA COMPLEX
A specific inflammatory condition of cats.

SIGNS
It causes red and inflamed swellings to develop on the skin
or mucous membranes of the mouth and throat, which
readily ulcerate. Eosinophilic ulcers on the lips are

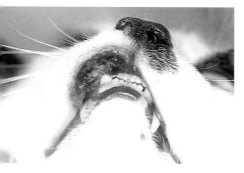

*Rodent
ulcer.*

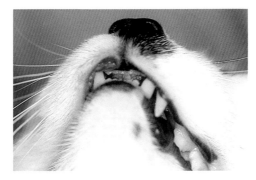

A rodent ulcer in the process of healing.

sometimes referred to as rodent ulcers, and can become cancerous if left untreated.

CAUSES
The cause is unknown, but it can be associated with chronic irritation, such as that associated with flea allergic dermatitis. This can cause eosinophilic granulomas to develop on the skin, where the cats licks excessively, or on the lip due to over-zealous grooming.

TREATMENT
If a source of irritation can be identified, such as fleas, it should be thoroughly treated. Indeed, intensive flea treatment is advisable for any cat with this condition. If it does not respond, then the use of anti-inflammatory drugs to control the problem is often needed.

EPILEPSY
See fits, page 179.

FELINE DYSAUTONOMIA

Originally known as the Key-Gaskell syndrome after the scientists that first described the disease in 1982, this disease causes a paralysis of the autonomic nervous system, the system which is responsible for controlling unconscious body functions such as digestion and bladder function. The strange thing about this condition is that it suddenly arrived in the United Kingdom in the 1980s, became quite a common condition, but gradually reduced in frequency until it is now rare.

SIGNS

Signs of the disease include dilation of the pupil, even in bright light, vomiting, constipation, depression and dehydration.

CAUSES

Despite intensive efforts to try and identify the cause, it has remained a complete mystery.

TREATMENT

Only symptomatic treatment can be given, and although many cats have died from the disease, it seems to be much milder when it does occur nowadays.

FELINE INFECTIOUS ANAEMIA (FIA)

A parasitic infection of the blood cells that results in their destruction, leading on to anaemia, a deficiency of circulating red blood cells (see anaemia, page 131).

SIGNS

The disease is most common in young cats, causing weakness and lethargy, with laboured breathing and collapse in severe cases. It may be possible to detect a pallor of the mucous membranes such as the gums, and a blood smear will demonstrate the parasite attached to the red blood cells. Some animals may suffer from infection without any signs of illness, which is often brought about by concurrent infection with another agent such as feline leukaemia virus. The disease often waxes and wanes. At some periods in its course the parasite cannot be found on blood smears, only to multiply again when the cat is stressed.

CAUSES
FIA is caused by infection with a single-celled organism called Haemobartonella felis. It is not proven how it is transmitted from cat to cat, but as the disease is more common in males, it is suspected that bites incurred during fighting may be a possible means, as well as being transmitted by blood-sucking parasites such as fleas.

TREATMENT
It can be very difficult to clear this disease completely, but a long course of treatment with an antibiotic such as oxytetracycline will at least help to bring about a remission.

FELINE INFECTIOUS ENTERITIS
See feline panleucopaenia, page 175.

FELINE INFECTIOUS PERITONITIS (FIP)
A viral disease of cats.

SIGNS
FIP is transmitted via the faeces and saliva, and is particularly common in multi-cat households. It is highly infectious, but only a small proportion of cats that come into contact with the virus actually develop the disease, and therefore a large number of cats will show positive for the virus on a blood test, yet not be suffering any ill effects.

The disease infectious peritonitis can take two forms – wet or dry –and occurs in young and middle-aged cats. The former is the most common, and results in an accumulation of a viscous amber fluid in the body cavities such as the abdomen and the chest, leading on to breathing difficulties and/or a distension of the abdomen.

In the dry form of the disease, multiple soft-tissue swellings develop on the linings of the body cavities, including around the brain, often resulting in neurological signs such as abnormal behaviour, blindness, and even convulsions. This is a very difficult disease to diagnose while the cat is still alive, and is one of the more common reasons for a cat being chronically unwell without any identifiable cause.

CAUSES
The condition is caused by infection with feline coronavirus. The most common result of infection with feline coronavirus is a relatively mild and self-limiting bout of diarrhoea. It was formerly thought that this was due to a separate strain of the virus, but this is now disputed, and it is thought to be the host's reaction to the infection that determines the form of disease that may result.

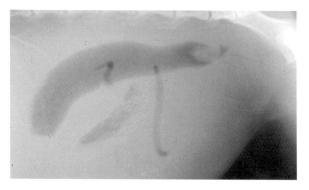

X-ray showing accumulation of fluid in the abdomen.

TREATMENT
A vaccine against the disease is available in the United States, but it only results in about a two-thirds reduction in the chance of contracting the disease. The vaccine is not available in the United Kingdom at the time of writing.

It is a generally a chronic, debilitating disease that, unfortunately, does not show much response to any form of treatment and always eventually leads to death. Drawing off the fluid is useful as a help in the diagnosis of the problem, but only results in a very short-term amelioration of the clinical signs as it rapidly accumulates again.

FELINE LEPROSY
A rare skin condition affecting cats, that is not related to leprosy in humans.

SIGNS
Single or multiple, frequently ulcerated and discharging nodules on the head or limbs.

CAUSES
Caused by a bacterium that is thought to be contracted by bites from rodents such as rats.

TREATMENT
Medical treatment is difficult, but surgical removal of the nodules may cure the problem.

FELINE LEUKAEMIA VIRUS (FeLV)
A virus that can infect cats and cause a range of problems including tumour development.

SIGNS
This virus can affect the immune system of the cat to cause an AIDS-like syndrome, where the cat's body is less able to defend itself against attack from infection. It can also attack the red blood-cells, causing severe anaemia, infertility, or cancers of the white blood-cells, often a considerable time after the original exposure to the virus. This can result in leukaemia, a cancer of the white blood-cells circulating in the blood stream, or lymphosarcoma, a cancer of the white blood-cells within the lymphatic tissue around the body. The clinical signs that develop will depend upon whereabouts within the body these growths develop, but the lymph nodes within the chest in young cats and in the intestines of older cats are particularly common sites.

CAUSES
The virus is spread by fairly close contact via saliva and faeces and is an important cause of ill health and death, particularly in young cats. A survey carried out across the UK in 1992 showed that about 10 per cent of all apparently healthy cats were infected with the virus. A cat that becomes infected may be able to expel the virus from their body entirely, the infection may become latent, which means that it lies dormant within the bone marrow, or the cat may become persistently infected with the virus in its blood. The latter is a serious problem for the cat, as the great majority will succumb to FeLV-related diseases and die within two years.

TREATMENT
At present, there is no drug that has proven to be effective in killing the virus without unacceptable side-effects, once

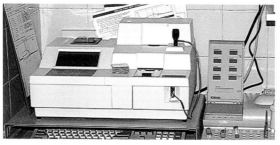

A blood analysis machine.

it has infected the cat. The research that has been carried out to date has led us to believe that the virus is not transmissible to humans.

The disease is readily diagnosed by means of a blood test, although a cat that proves positive on an initial blood screening test should be re-tested after six weeks to see if it has managed to eliminate the virus from its blood. It is essential that any cats introduced to a closed breeding colony or brought for mating to a stud tom are blood-tested beforehand to ensure they are not a carrier.

Vaccines against FeLV have become available during the 1990s, and have proven themselves to be safe and effective. The vaccination of young cats against FeLV at the same time as the vaccine given for cat flu and feline panleucopaenia virus is now becoming routine, and is strongly advisable.

FELINE PANLEUCOPAENIA
This was the first feline disease to be proven to be caused by a virus, and consequently the first for which a vaccine became available. It used to be called feline distemper or feline infectious enteritis.

SIGNS
The virus attacks the white blood cells and the lining of the intestine, causing acute diarrhoea and often death within three or four days of the onset of illness. It is a very resistant virus that can survive for many months in the environment, and is passed on in the faeces or other body discharges. This disease was once called 'feline distemper', and although it bears no relation to the virus that causes canine distemper, it is closely related to the parvovirus that causes severe diarrhoea in dogs. If a pregnant queen becomes infected and survives, the kittens may be affected by 'feline ataxia', a

wobbly gait due to brain damage caused by the virus.

CAUSES
The virus that causes the disease is passed in large quantities
in the faeces of sick cats and can remain in the environment
for many months. It is also resistant to many disinfectants.

TREATMENT
This disease has been a fine example of the effectiveness of
a vaccination programme, as the vaccine that was developed
in the 1970s has proven to give a solid protection against the
disease and to be extremely safe. From being a disease that
was a relatively common cause of severe illness in cats, it is
now seen only rarely, and then only in areas where there are
a large number of unvaccinated cats. A live feline
panleucopaenia vaccine can protect a cat for two years or
more, although it is now generally given annually in the all-
in-one booster vaccinations.

FELINE SPONGIFORM
ENCEPHALOPATHY (FSE)
**Also called 'mad cat disease', this is a disorder of the
nervous system of cats that was first recognised in the
United Kingdom in April 1990. Only one other case has
been seen in a domestic cat outside the UK. That was in
Norway.**

SIGNS
Primary signs of the disease involve an alteration in normal
behaviour, including a loss of balance, increased sensitivity
to sound and touch, and a strange gait.

CAUSES
Changes seen post-mortem in the brain of affected cats
suggest that it is caused by the same agent that causes BSE,
or 'mad cow disease', and it is presumed that cats have
caught the disease by eating offal from infected cows.
Fortunately, the Pet Food Manufacturers Association in the
UK voluntarily banned the use of offals that were thought to
be likely to pass on the disease in 1988, a ban that became
a legal requirement in 1990. The condition has remained
rare in cats, reaching a peak of 16 reported cases in 1994,
falling to 8 in 1995 and just one in the first half of 1996.

TREATMENT
The condition is invariably fatal once clinical signs develop,

and has to be reported by a veterinary surgeon to the Ministry of Agriculture.

FELINE TUBERCULOSIS
Infection with one of the Mycobacterium group of bacteria.

SIGNS
The most common form of the disease appears as skin lumps that sometimes burst to leave open sores, especially on the cat's face and legs. Only a few cases of this disease are diagnosed each year, and unlike the other forms of TB, it is not transmissible to humans.

CAUSES
It is possible for cats to catch tuberculosis (TB) from humans and develop similar signs of lung disease, but thankfully the low incidence of the human disease means that this is extremely rare. Similarly, bovine tuberculosis has almost been eradicated from many national herds, so cats no longer commonly contract this form of the disease by drinking infected milk. Recent studies have shown that some cases of skin disease in cats are due to a more unusual strain of the bacterium, and it is thought that this is contracted from wild rodents such as voles, which, of course, would be a common prey species in the rural areas where this disease can occur.

TREATMENT
Treatment for several weeks with special anti-TB drugs can cure the skin problem.

FELINE UROLOGICAL SYNDROME (FUS)
An accumulation of fine crystals within the bladder and urethra.

SIGNS
Straining, discomfort, sometimes bleeding into the urine, and, in male cats, possibly complete obstruction of the urethra so that the cat is unable to urinate. This is only likely to occur in males because in females the urethra is much wider and the debris can be passed.

CAUSES

It is not known exactly why some cats develop FUS, but it is clear that diet plays a major part. The crystals that form are usually based upon a substance called struvite, which is a crystalline compound of magnesium that tends to form in an alkaline urine.

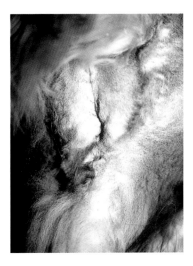

Perineal urethrostomy.

TREATMENT

A diet that is low in magnesium and produces an acidic urine can play a major role in treating and preventing recurrence in susceptible cats, but it is not known why one cat develops the problem on a normal complete feline diet whereas another may not.

Surveys have shown that the problem is more common in cats that are neutered, overweight, and not very active – although, of course, these factors could well be linked to each other! It is vital that the owner of a male cat realises that if their cat is straining to urinate and in obvious distress, it could be suffering from a urinary blockage and needs immediate veterinary attention to avoid serious damage to the bladder and kidneys.

Cats with a blockage obviously need to have it cleared and to have a urinary catheter put into place under anaesthetic. If the obstruction cannot be cleared, or the urethra keeps blocking up again when the catheter is removed, a permanent by-pass operation, called a perineal urethrotomy, may be performed. This piece of plastic surgery reshapes the lower part of the male urethra to resemble that of the female.

Medical treatment of FUS mainly involves a change of diet to a complete pre-prepared food that is low in magnesium and produces an acidic urine – there are several on the market in both canned and dry form. Antibiotics are often given to prevent secondary infection, and although bacteria cannot usually be cultured from the urine, antibiotics often seem to help alleviate the discomfort.

Cats that suffer from repeated bouts of lower urinary problems are usually X-rayed to rule out other problems, such as large calculi (stones) that may form within the bladder, and tumours of the bladder wall, which are sometimes seen in older cats.

FELINE VIRAL RHINOTRACHEITIS

This virus is a herpesvirus, and like other herpesviruses (such as the one that causes cold sores in humans), it can lie dormant in the nerve tissue of the body, and become active when the host's resistance is low.

SIGNS
One of the major causes of cat flu (see page 146), it results in conjunctivitis, runny nose, sneezing, and general ill health. In rare cases, it can cause ulcers to develop on the surface of the eye (cornea).

CAUSES
The infection is passed from cat to cat, generally by sneezing.

TREATMENT
Modern cat flu vaccines give good protection against this organism, but once infected, only supportive treatment can be given while the cat's immune system fights off the virus. Topical antiviral drops can be used in cases of corneal ulceration.

FITS

A temporary but sudden loss of consciousness, accompanied by severe involuntary contractions of the

jaw and body muscles. Also known as convulsions or seizures.

SIGNS
Fits can vary in intensity, but generally cause the cat to fall on to its side, extend its legs, and arch its back, accompanied by profuse salivation and paddling of the limbs. The eyes remain open, breathing is rapid, and the cat may pass urine and faeces. This may last for up to five minutes, and is usually followed by a period of depression and confusion, sometimes with the cat showing temporary neurological signs such as apparent blindness. Very mild fits may only last a matter of seconds.

CAUSES
Many physical abnormalities can trigger off the electrical activity in the brain that causes the fit, such as liver disease, kidney disease, infections such as feline infectious peritonitis or the ingestion of some form of poison. Problems within the brain itself, such as injury, infection or tumours, can also cause fits to develop. A cat that has a fit will require investigations to rule out any underlying cause, but sometimes the fits can be due to idiopathic epilepsy, which mainly affects young cats and is thought to be inherited.

TREATMENT
It is best not to disturb a cat while it is having a fit – just make sure it is out of harm's way, preferably in a dark and quiet room, and keep it under close observation. If the fit lasts for more than about five minutes, or if the cat keeps having fits in quick succession, then urgent veterinary attention is required.

Once a fit has subsided, a careful clinical examination and possibly blood tests will be required to try and establish the cause. Some underlying problems may be treatable, and, of course, any harmful substances that may have affected the cat should be put well out of reach. A brain tumour can be treated with the use of a scanner to identify the mass. Surgery may be necessary to remove it – but this is only available in one or two very specialised referral centres at considerable cost. Some cases require longterm treatment with anticonvulsants such as phenobarbitone to control the problem.

FLEAS

Fleas are wingless blood-sucking insects that live on their host most of the time. They lay their eggs on the ground, where they develop into larvae which feed upon organic debris such as the faeces of the adult flea and dry flakes of skin from the cat. They then form pupae, which can lie dormant for many months, and hatch out as a response to vibrations and carbon dioxide produced by their new host.

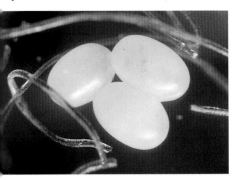

Flea eggs.

SIGNS

Some cats carry a considerable number of fleas without any visible problem, but owners may notice the rapidly-moving fleas themselves, or more likely, the dark-coloured flea dirt. These are the fleas' droppings, consisting mainly of undigested blood, and may be seen either on the cat itself, or on its bedding. Flea dirt can easily be distinguished from grit by putting it on to some damp cotton wool – a reddish halo will be seen around it as the blood dissolves in the moisture. Fleas are by far the most important cause of skin problems in cats (see allergic dermatitis, page 126). They may also transmit other diseases such as feline infectious anaemia (page 171) and tapeworm (page 239).

CAUSES

Cat fleas are picked up directly from other cats or dogs, or more commonly, by passing through areas which have been infested with eggs that have developed in to pupae that are ready to hatch out and hop on to a new host. Just occasionally, cats will be infested with other fleas, such as the dog, rabbit or hedgehog flea, but the cat flea is by far the most common. Fleas are an increasing problem as they thrive in the warm, poorly-ventilated conditions that we provide for them all year round in our homes.

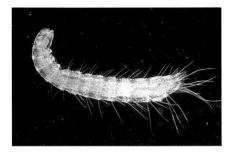

Flea larvae.

Flea dirt seen on a cat's coat.

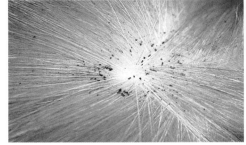

TREATMENT

Prevention is better than cure. It is possible to use an insecticide on a regular basis, but it is preferable to use a product that prevents the fleas from developing. This is available as a veterinary prescription product under the trade name of Program, and is given as a liquid once a month – dogs in the home must also be treated with the drug in tablet form. This is an extremely safe product that makes any fleas that bite a treated cat infertile, so that they die out within a week or two without establishing an infestation around the house.

If adult fleas are seen, an insecticide should be used on all cats and dogs in the house. Shampoos only have a very short-acting effect and are not easy to use in the cat, and collars are not, in my experience, very safe or effective. Drop-on products are now quite widely used, as a small amount of liquid only has to be dropped on to the back of the neck once a month. Although they are easy to use, the instructions for safe administration must be followed closely.

The most modern generation of insecticides such as fipronil (available on veterinary prescription under the trade name Frontline) are much safer than many of the older preparations, very effective, and long-lasting (up to two months in the case of Frontline). Many owners have

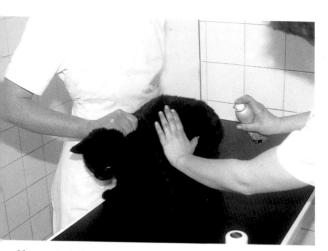

If a cat is infested with fleas, it will need to be sprayed with an insecticide.

problems with using an aerosol spray on their cats, but may find it easier to wear a disposable plastic glove, spray the insecticide on to the glove, and then rub it into the coat.

It is essential to understand that once an infestation has established itself, the environment must be treated as well as the pet. Sprays and powders are available, and it is even possible to call in the local authority or a private company to thoroughly fumigate the house. Your veterinary surgeon should be able to offer you the best advice on all aspects of flea control.

FOREIGN BODIES

A term used to describe any item that is not normally present in the body, but gains entry and causes a problem. This could include objects such as grass awns

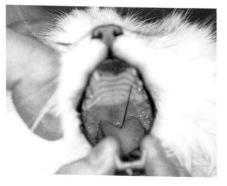

Foreign body: a needle in the mouth.

183

in the ear or back of the throat, small particles in the eye, or indigestible substances that have been swallowed but are unable to pass through the digestive tract. See chronic rhinitis (page 149), ear disease (page 166), keratitis (page 202, vomiting (page 247).

FRACTURES

A partial or complete break in the normal structure of the bone. The fracture is more serious if the bone breaks the skin, which could allow infection to enter.

SIGNS
A fractured bone will cause a deformity, pain, and also swelling and warmth at the site of the break. It may even be possible to feel a grating of the broken ends of the bone against each other.

CAUSES
Generally as a result of accidental injury such as a fall or a road accident, although pathological fractures can occur with very minimal trauma if the bones are weakened due to some other underlying condition such as kidney disease, poor nutrition, or a bone tumour.

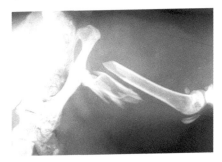

A fractured femur.

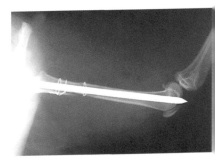

Repair of a fractured femur.

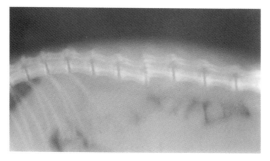

A fractured spine.

TREATMENT

An owner should not attempt to manipulate or splint a broken bone, as further damage can easily be caused, and the prognosis is much worse if a sharp piece of bone penetrates the skin and infection enters the fracture site. A vet's first priority is to treat any life-threatening injuries and allow the cat to recover from the shock of the injury, before carrying out radiography of the fracture and any necessary treatment.

A fractured jaw.

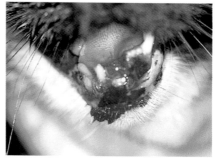

Fractures of the limb extremities may be treated with a cast, although synthetic ones are now more commonly used than plaster of Paris, as they are lighter and stronger. Cats are not very tolerant of casts, and all but the most minor of fractures are usually treated by internal fixation, where metal pins, plates, wire and screws are used to stabilise the fracture and allow a rapid return to normal movement.

GANGRENE
Death and decay of body tissue.

SIGNS
Gangrenous tissue will usually become moist and foul-smelling, causing the cat considerable discomfort. Eventually, toxins released into the body will make the cat very unwell.

CAUSES
Damage to the blood supply to a part of the body, such as severe injury to the tail or a limb, or when a dressing is applied too tightly.

TREATMENT
If the cause of the problem can be rectified, then it obviously must be carried out quickly, before irreversible damage results. Antibiotics can be used to control the spread of infection while the dead tissue sloughs off, but in severe cases it must be surgically removed, which may involve amputation of a limb (see amputation, page 129).

GASTRO-ENTERITIS
Gastritis is an inflammation of the stomach and is often accompanied by enteritis, an inflammation of the intestines. For details of specific causes, see under diarrhoea (page 163) and vomiting (page 247).

GIARDIASIS
We are just beginning to appreciate the importance of this tiny parasite in causing diarrhoea in cats.

SIGNS
This disease is a relatively common, though often undiagnosed, cause of chronic diarrhoea, causing loose or watery motions, sometimes with mucus (see diarrhoea page 163).

CAUSES
A single-celled parasite called giardia, that is passed by

faecal contamination from cat to cat, particularly in conditions of poor hygiene or overcrowded housing. The organism can be identified in a stool sample examined under the microscope, although sometimes multiple samples have to be examined as the organism is only shed intermittently.

TREATMENT
A course of a specific antibiotic called metronidazole can be used to cure this condition.

GINGIVITIS
An inflammation of the gums that is often combined with a more generalised inflammation of the mouth, known as stomatitis.

SIGNS
This is a very common condition in cats, and can be seen as a reddening of the gums and other tissues of the mouth. This can lead to signs of oral discomfort, such as difficulty in eating, excess salivation, and pawing at the mouth, as well as bad breath and bleeding from the gums.

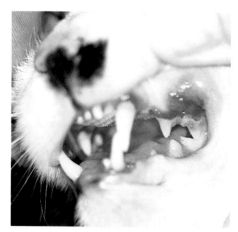

Gingivitis due to tartar accumulation.

CAUSES
There are a large number of possible causes of this condition, but it is most commonly associated with tooth problems (see dental disease, page 159). Other causes include viral infections such as feline calicivirus, feline leukaemia virus and feline immunodeficiency virus, direct

irritation from caustic agents that are either chewed or groomed off the coat, and more generalised disease such as kidney failure and diabetes mellitus. Idiopathic chronic stomatitis is a term applied to a long-standing inflammation of the oral cavity where no underlying cause can be identified, and this is not uncommon in cats.

TREATMENT
Any underlying disease needs appropriate treatment, particularly the removal of dental calculus and extraction of any teeth causing significant problems. Whatever the underlying cause, the inflammation is often complicated by bacterial infection, and treatment with antibiotics may be needed. Some cases require long-term control with anti-inflammatory drugs such as prednisolone.

GLAUCOMA
An increase in pressure of the fluid within the eyeball.

SIGNS
Reddening of the tissues around the eye, pain, clouding of the cornea at the front of the eye, dilation of the pupil and behavioural signs of blindness if both eyes are affected. An enlargement of the globe of one eye compared to the other may also be visible.

CAUSES
This is not a common condition in cats, and usually develops secondarily to some other condition that causes inflammation within the eye and blocks the drainage of fluid out from the eyeball.

TREATMENT
Drug treatment and, possibly, surgery to help drain fluid from the eyeball can sometimes help. However, all too often permanent blindness results, and in some cases the affected eye has to be removed to provide relief from long-term pain.

GLOMERULONEPHRITIS
See nephrotic syndrome, page 213.

GLOSSITIS
An inflammation of the tongue, usually associated with a more generalised inflammation of the mouth (see stomatitis, page 238).

HAEMOPHILIA

A hereditary blood disorder causing a failure of normal blood clotting, so that an affected animal bleeds excessively from even a minor wound. It is not common in cats.

HAEMORRHAGE

A loss of blood, either externally, with obvious blood loss to the outside, or internally within the body.

SIGNS
External bleeding is obvious, but internal bleeding into the abdomen or chest may be much harder to detect. The loss of red blood cells will cause laboured breathing, weakness, and paleness of the normally pink mucous membranes such as the gums.

CAUSES
Injuries such as road accidents, tumours, and poisoning with drugs that affect the clotting of the blood (see warfarin poisoning, page 249).

TREATMENT
First Aid measures should be taken to staunch the flow of blood (See First Aid and Nursing, page 90), but detecting and treating the underlying cause of internal bleeding can be difficult. Mild internal bleeding may cease and the blood become reabsorbed into the body, but where there is severe or prolonged bleeding, it may be necessary to consider a blood transfusion from another cat as a life-saving procedure.

HAIR BALLS

It is normal for a cat to vomit up small amounts of hair that has been swallowed during the grooming process, but sometimes an excessive accumulation of hair can cause problems.

SIGNS
A build-up of hair within the stomach may put the cat off its food due to the distension that it causes. The cat may also vomit repeatedly, yet be unable to clear the hair.

CAUSES
This condition is particularly common in long-haired cats, especially if they are not groomed regularly by their owners.

TREATMENT
A laxative such as liquid paraffin will act as a lubricant and may help the hair to pass through, and regular grooming will often prevent the problem from occurring in the first place. If the cat does not improve within a day or two, veterinary attention should be sought to rule out any other possible causes.

HEATSTROKE
Cats are descended from desert-living ancestors, and can adapt very well to high environment temperatures. Therefore, compared to animals such as dogs, they very rarely suffer from heatstroke, unless exposed to the most extreme conditions.

SIGNS
Panting, weakness, and finally collapse.

CAUSES
Prolonged exposure to high environmental temperatures, such as inside a car in hot and sunny weather.

TREATMENT
Immediate bathing in cool water to get the body temperature down, followed by prompt veterinary assistance. Intravenous fluid replacement therapy is usually necessary.

HAEMOTHORAX
The presence of free blood within the chest cavity.

SIGNS
Rapid heart rate and respiration with pallor of the mucous membranes and sometimes collapse.

CAUSES
Usually associated with severe trauma such as a road

accident. It can also be caused by bleeding tumours within the chest, or blood clotting disorders. An X-ray is usually necessary to confirm the diagnosis, and possibly thoracocentesis – the drawing off of fluid from the chest.

TREATMENT
Mild cases will usually resolve with strict rest, but fluid therapy may be necessary to support the circulation due to blood loss. Rapid or continuous bleeding may require an exploratory operation to determine the cause, but the surgical risks are very high.

HEART DISEASE
Unlike humans, who most commonly suffer from disease of the coronary arteries, and dogs, that most commonly suffer from disease of the heart valves, cats most commonly suffer from disease of the heart muscle itself, a condition known as cardiomyopathy.

SIGNS
The main sign shown by a cat with cardiomyopathy is laboured respiration caused by a build-up of fluid on the lungs, as well as lethargy and lack of appetitie. Some cats suddenly become paralysed in their hind legs due to a blood clot forming in the main arteries, resulting from the poor circulation (see iliac thrombosis page). A radiograph of the heart will often diagnose the heart problem, although fluid may have to be drawn off the lungs before a diagnostic X-ray can be taken. A referral centre may use more specialised techniques such as an electrocardiograph to measure the

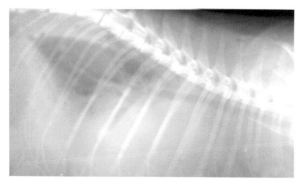

X-ray of cat suffering from cardiomyopathy.

electrical activity of the heart, an echocardiograph to record the heart sounds, and ultrasound, which can make visible the flow of blood through the heart.

CAUSES
The condition is caused by a degeneration in the heart muscle itself (as opposed to disease of the heart valves, which is by far the commonest condition in the dog). It can take two forms – dilated cardiomyopathy, where the heart muscle becomes weak and dilated, and hypertrophic cardiomyopathy, where the heart muscle becomes greatly thickened and loses its ability to expand and contract properly.

Dilated cardiomyopathy used to be quite a common condition, until it was discovered that the major cause of the problem is a deficiency of an amino acid called taurine in the diet. Although the vast majority of cats were able to manage perfectly well on the levels previously recommended in commercial cat foods, some cats seemed to have a higher requirement than others. Since this has been discovered, the manufacturers of cat foods have boosted the levels of taurine in their diets. As a result, the incidence of the problem has been greatly reduced – to the point where it is only likely to be seen in cats eating very poor-quality commercial or home-made diets.

Hypertrophic cardiomyopathy can develop when a cat suffers from chronically high blood pressure, although this cannot easily be measured. An overactive thyroid (see hyperthyroidism, page 195) is one of the major causes of the condition, although in many cases no underlying cause can be found.

About 2 per cent of cats are born with a congenital heart disorder, ranging in severity from those that show no clinical signs through their life, to those that die of the problem soon after birth. Affected cats tend to grow less quickly than others in the litter, they tire quickly and may develop breathing difficulties.

TREATMENT
If an underlying problem causing cardiomyopathy, such as an overactive thyroid or a dietary deficiency, can be corrected, then the long-term outlook for the cat is quite good, but often the best that can be achieved is permanent drug treatment to try and control the problem, including the use of anticoagulants to try and prevent unwanted blood clots from forming. The life expectancy for a cat with

severe congenital heart disease is poor, but surgical correction can sometimes be attempted.

HEPATITIS
See liver disease, page 206.

HERNIA
A weakness or unusual opening in the body wall that can lead to the protrusion of fat or of an internal organ.

SIGNS
The commonest types of hernia in the cat are umbilical (where the belly-button is), inguinal (in the groin) and incisional (through a previous operation scar, usually in the midline of the abdomen). They cause an abnormal soft swelling that fluctuates if the herniated tissue is pushed back into the body. If this tissue becomes entrapped in the hernia and the blood supply is cut off, the hernia is said to be strangulated, and will become inflamed and tender.

CAUSES
Most hernias are hereditary, although an umbilical hernia can be caused if the queen tears off the umbilical cord from the kitten very roughly. An incisional hernia is due to poor healing of a surgical wound.

TREATMENT
Small hernias can be left untreated, or repaired when a cat has a general anaesthetic for some other reason, such as neutering. Larger ones may need repair more urgently, using a technique known as herniorrhaphy. Strangulated hernias constitute an acute emergency if a vital organ has become entrapped.

HOOKWORMS
A parasite that attaches to the lining of the small intestine and sucks blood.

SIGNS
Severe anaemia leading to weakness and emaciation.

CAUSES
A worm called Ancyclostomum. It is found in tropical and sub-tropical countries, and is extremely rare in the UK.

TREATMENT
Regular worming with a preparation effective against hookworms in areas where it is known to occur.

HORNER'S SYNDROME
A particular pattern of clinical signs caused by damage to one of the many nerves controlling the eye and its lids.

SIGNS
A retraction of the eyeball, a drooping of the eyelid and a contraction of the pupil on the affected side.

CAUSES
It is due to damage to the nerve that controls a particular group of muscles to the eye and the iris. This nerve passes along the neck and by the base of the ear before it reaches the eye, so it is prone to injury especially if the cat is involved in a road accident, or if there is an infection in the deeper parts of the ear.

TREATMENT
Any ear problem will need appropriate treatment, but the nerve damage almost always recovers with time.

HYPERADRENOCORTICALISM
Also known as Cushing's syndrome, it is due to an excessive production of cortisone by the adrenal glands, which are situated just above each kidney.

SIGNS
This condition is being recognised with increasing frequency in middle-aged and older cats, causing increased thirst and appetite. The high levels of cortisone in the blood tend to cause the cat to develop diabetes mellitus (see page 161), and this syndrome is the commonest cause of diabetes mellitus that fails to respond adequately to insulin treatment.

CAUSES
The disease can be caused either by a tumour of the pituitary gland at the base of the brain, that produces another hormone called ACTH that in turn controls the level of cortisone production by the adrenal glands, or by a tumour of an adrenal gland itself. This can be confirmed by a blood test to measure cortisone levels in the blood before and after an injection of ACTH.

TREATMENT
Surgical removal of excess adrenal gland tissue.

HYPERPARATHYROIDISM

An over-production of parathyroid hormone by the parathyroid glands, which are closely attached to each of the two thyroid glands in the neck. This hormone controls calcium levels in the body.

SIGNS
Weakening of the bones due to removal of calcium from the bone tissue, causing lameness and possibly even spontaneous fractures.

CAUSES
This condition is most commonly seen in kittens, due to feeding a meat and cereal based diet that is high in phosphorus and low in calcium. In older cats, the condition may develop due to a problem with calcium balance that can occur in cats with chronic kidney disease.

TREATMENT
Correction of dietary levels of calcium and phosphorus, and treatment of any underlying kidney problem, if appropriate.

HYPERTHYROIDISM

An over-production of thyroid hormone. It was first recognised in 1979, but is now very frequently diagnosed.

SIGNS
Cats have two thyroid glands, situated on either side of the lower neck region, that in a normal cat cannot be felt externally. The hormone that they produce regulates the metabolic rate of the body – the rate at which it burns up energy. Therefore a cat with hyperthyroidism becomes very hyperactive and all its bodily functions take place too rapidly. The affected cat will drink excessively, eat constantly, yet lose weight. Vomiting and, more particularly, diarrhoea are often associated with the condition. Respiratory and heart rates are more rapid than normal, leading to heart failure if untreated.

The heart problems that develop may, in turn, cause blood clots to form in places such as the arteries to the leg, causing sudden paralysis of the hindlimbs (see iliac thrombosis page

198). An enlarged gland may be felt in the neck region, but a blood test is needed to confirm the diagnosis. If the cat is unwell, this can sometimes lower the blood thyroid levels leading to a normal result in a cat that does, in fact, have an overactive gland, and so more than one test may be necessary.

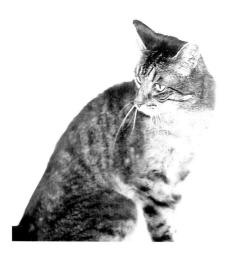

A hyperthyroid cat.

CAUSES

The condition is due to a tumour in one or both thyroid glands. Although the growths are not usually cancerous, they produce a wide range of physical problems if they excrete excessive amounts of hormone into the blood. It is the commonest hormonal condition affecting cats and a major cause of disease in elderly cats. It has been suggested that the problem may be sparked off by some environmental factor, but this is as yet unproven. Although dogs quite commonly suffer from an under-active thyroid, this is thought to be extremely rare in the cat.

TREATMENT

There are currently three options for treatment. Drugs are available that can lower the blood thyroid levels, but they have to be given twice a day on a permanent basis and can sometimes cause untoward side-effects. An operation to remove one or both thyroid glands is commonly performed and usually has very good results – although cats are often put on to drug treatment first to reduce the strain on the heart from the effects of the excess thyroid hormone before an anaesthetic is given. Although cats can usually manage perfectly well without their thyroid glands, there is a very small gland called the parathyroid quite closely attached to the thyroid gland. The parathyroid controls calcium balance within the body, and a cat cannot survive without at least one functioning parathyroid gland, so great care has to be taken to try and leave them undamaged when the thyroids are removed. Even cats that have had both thyroid glands removed surgically often seem to be able to cope without any additional hormone supplementation.

The third treatment is rather more dramatic, although it is possibly the ideal, as it does not involve any surgery yet results in a permanent cure. The cat is injected with radioactive iodine that is taken up by the thyroid and destroys the gland. The only problem is that the cat then becomes radioactive for several weeks, and has to be kept in isolation. This treatment is only available in a few specially licensed centres.

Whichever form of treatment is selected, the condition can usually be very successfully treated, and even a very old and frail cat may be given a very useful extra lease of life.

HYPERVITAMINOSIS A
While cats can suffer from a deficiency of vitamin A if their diet is very low in the vitamin, it is much more common for them to suffer illness due to an excess.

SIGNS
An excess of vitamin A in the diet affects bone formation, causing lameness, stiffness of the joints (especially the vertebral joints of the neck) and pain. An X-ray will show up large amounts of new bone formation around the body.

CAUSES
Feeding an unbalanced diet, particularly an excess of liver, which is very rich in vitamin A. Many cats are very fond of eating liver, and can easily become 'hooked' on it if their owners allow. Cod-liver oil also contains large amounts of vitamin A, and this condition can be caused by over-zealous supplementation.

TREATMENT
Correction of the diet and anti-inflammatory drugs, but permanent disability often results.

ILIAC THROMBOSIS
A sudden blockage due to a blood clot in the arterial blood supply to the hind legs.

SIGNS
The cat suddenly becomes completely paralysed in its hind legs, with the legs either going completely limp, or becoming very stiff and immobile. The condition is very painful, and the cat is often in considerable distress.

CAUSES
The clot usually forms because the blood is not circulating properly due to cardiomyopathy (see page 145), and this in turn is most commonly due to an over-active thyroid gland (see hyperthyroidism, page 195).

TREATMENT
Euthanasia may be the kindest course of action in view of the likelihood of an underlying heart condition, and because the cat is likely to be in considerable pain. Affected cats given pain-killing drugs will usually recover the use of the limbs with time, and anti-clotting drugs can be given to try and prevent recurrence. Surgical removal of the clot has been attempted, but the survival rate is not good.

INFERTILITY
A failure to reproduce, which can be due to problems with the queen or the tom.

CAUSES
In the male, infertility is usually either due to a reluctance to mate, which is quite common in young toms, or due to poor sperm production. The causes in the female are rather more complex, and can affect any stage of the process:-
Failure to call – some queens, particularly certain pedigree cats such as Persians, mature very late in life. Timid queens housed in a group with other entire females may suppress the signs of oestrus. Hormonal disorders also occur, but are very difficult to identify and treat.

Failure to mate – uncommon, but may be seen in nervous queens that travel to a stud tom and are not allowed time to settle down before mating.

Failure to conceive – hormonal imbalances may prevent the queen from ovulating normally, or prevent the fertilised egg from implanting in the womb. Sometimes there is even a physical abnormality, with an essential part of the reproductive tract missing.

Failure to carry kittens to full term – this is the most common cause of infertility, where the foetuses are conceived, but are either resorbed back into the body or aborted. This is most often due to an infection that affects the reproductive tract, particularly with feline leukaemia virus. Chronic endometritis is a thickening of the lining of the womb, often with secondary bacterial infection, that causes a vaginal discharge and frequently leads to infertility.

Failure to give birth – much less common in queens than in bitches, but this can be due to excessively large litters over-stretching the womb, a very small litter not stimulating the womb to contract properly, or a large or deformed kitten obstructing the birth canal.

TREATMENT

Murphy's Law of veterinary science dictates that a valuable queen that goes to a stud tom to be mated may well not give birth to kittens, whereas if she escapes out of the back door and mates with the neighbourhood beau she will fall pregnant immediately! There is some doubt as to whether cats that have major problems conceiving should be given extensive treatment to cure the problem, as they in all likelihood in turn produce kittens that go on to have similar problems. As always, if the cause of the problem can be determined and corrected, a cure may be effected. Caesarean section is quite commonly carried out in cats that are unable to give birth, but again, repeated mating of such cats is usually inadvisable.

INTUSSUSCEPTION

A condition where a section of the intestine rolls up on itself, rather like the finger of a rubber glove when it is pulled off the hand, causing a complete or partial obstruction to the passage of food.

SIGNS

This is an uncommon condition; however, it is most

commonly seen in young cats with diarrhoea, and may lead to straining, abdominal pain, vomiting, and death if left untreated. A veterinary surgeon may be able to feel the sausage-shaped mass within the abdomen, but an X-ray is necessary to confirm the diagnosis.

CAUSES
It is not known why some cats develop this condition.

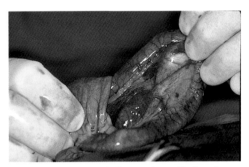

Surgery is required if a cat is suffering from intussusception.

TREATMENT
Once diagnosed, an immediate operation is necessary to either unroll the obstruction, or more commonly, to remove the length of bowel that has been affected and suture the remaining ends back together again. Although this shortens the length of bowel, most cats can adjust to this and return to normal.

J

JAUNDICE
A yellowness of the tissues due to the accumulation of bile pigments in the body.

SIGNS
Yellowing of the skin, the mucous membranes (such as the gums) and the whites of the eyes. The cat has a lack of appetite and and is generally unwell.

CAUSES
Bile pigments are found in large quantities in the red blood cells, and when these cells become aged and are broken down in the body, the pigments are excreted via the liver, down the gall duct and into the faeces. A build-up of bile pigments can occur if excessive amounts of red blood cells are being destroyed (see anaemia, page 131), if the liver is diseased and unable to cope with processing the bile (see liver disease, page 206), or if there is an obstruction to the flow of bile out of the liver, such as by a tumour blocking the bile duct. Blood tests will help to determine the cause of the jaundice, which is a sign of ill health rather than a disease entity in itself.

TREATMENT
Once the underlying cause of the build-up of bile has been identified and corrected, the bile pigments will slowly be resorbed back from the tissues. However, this process can take many weeks.

KERATITIS
An inflammation of the cornea, the front 'window' of the eye.

SIGNS
Acute keratitis will cause pain, spasm of the pupil, a tendency to hold the eye shut, excessive tear production, redness of the eye, and a cloudiness of the normally clear cornea. In more long-standing cases, blood vessels may be seen to grow across the surface of the eye, and dark pigmentation may develop. In severe cases, ulceration of the superficial surface of the cornea may occur, and this may even completely penetrate into the eye, posing a major threat to the cat's vision in that eye. A green dye called fluoroscein can be put into the eye to show up any areas of ulceration (see corneal ulceration, page 153).

CAUSES
Common causes include scratches from other cats, foreign bodies in the eye, and infections.

TREATMENT
Antibiotics, possibly together with anti-inflammatory treatment in the form of drops or ointment are usually necessary. In severe cases of ulceration, it may be necessary to suture a portion of the conjunctiva over the lesion to protect it while it heals.

KIDNEY DISEASE
The kidneys are responsible for eliminating waste products from the body and maintaining fluid balance. Kidney disease is a very significant cause of illness in cats.

SIGNS
The first warning is an increased thirst due to an inability to concentrate the urine as efficiently, but as many cats do not drink from a bowl, this can be difficult to identify. An observant owner may notice a change in the cat's pattern of

behaviour, and a cat that perhaps never used to drink much at all, may be spotted regularly drinking from a pond, a tap or other water source.

As the disease process progresses, waste products from the breakdown of protein within the body start to build up, and, in turn, cause further damage to the remaining kidney tissue. Signs of kidney disease include:-

•Excessive thirst
•Lack of appetitie
•Weight Loss
•Poor condition
•Bad breath
•Ulcers in the mouth
•Softening of the bones
•Anaemia

Eventually, the cat will refuse to eat altogether. It may start to have convulsions, and will inevitably die.

Once the disease develops, a blood test will show an increase of urea in the blood, as well as an increase in an enzyme called creatinine. An increasing number of veterinary practices are using a combination of blood and urine tests during routine health screens of elderly pets to pick up impending problems at an early stage.

CAUSES

There are many possible causes of kidney disease, such as bacterial infections, congenital abnormalities, the effect of toxins, and tumours. However, by far the commonest cause is chronic interstitial nephritis – a gradual replacement of the normal kidney tissue with scar tissue, that develops with age.

The causes are not well understood, nor why some cats develop it much sooner than others. It is possible for the a cat to have up to two-thirds of its kidney filtration cells damaged without showing any signs of illness at all, so by the time that the condition is clinically recognisable, the underlying disease process is already well advanced.

TREATMENT

A lot can be done to slow down the progression of the disease and give the cat a longer lease of life, but early diagnosis is essential. If an underlying cause such as an infection can be identified, then, of course, it must be treated. However, most frequently we can only give palliative treatment to enable the cat to cope as well as possible with the kidney function that it has remaining. Cats are often dehydrated by the time the problem is diagnosed, so an intravenous drip may be needed to correct this. Drugs may also be used, such as vitamins and anabolic steroids to stimulate the appetite, and anti-emetics to control vomiting.

The most important aspect of treating kidney disease involves a change in diet to a food specially designed to reduce the work load on the kidneys. Cats cannot manage on very low protein diets, but a diet with a moderately restricted level of high-quality, easily digested protein will reduce the amount of protein waste products that build up in the body. Even more important is a restriction on the amount of phosphorus in the diet, as this accumulates in the body of cats with kidney problems and causes further damage to the kidneys.

The levels of B vitamins need to be boosted because they tend to be lost from the body when the kidneys are not working properly. While it is theoretically possible to achieve this with a home-made diet, it is extremely difficult to get the balance just right, and a range of pre-prepared diets are available from veterinary surgeries to help control the problem. See also nephrotic syndrome page 213.

KINKED TAIL
A common condition, particularly in Siamese cats, that is only of significance in show cats.

SIGNS
A kink near the end of the tail.

CAUSES
A hereditary deformity in the tail vertebrae.

TREATMENT
No treatment is necessary.

L

LACTATION TETANY

Also known as eclampsia, this is a rare complication of pregnancy in the cat.

SIGNS
Can occur during pregnancy itself, or while the queen is feeding the kittens. It causes restlessness, incoordination, muscle tremors, and progresses to fits if left untreated.

CAUSES
Low blood calcium levels due to the demands of the developing kittens.

TREATMENT
A veterinary surgeon needs to administer an injection of a calcium solution promptly to prevent the condition from getting worse.

LARYNGITIS

An inflammation of the larynx, or voicebox.

SIGNS
Dysphonia (loss or voice), retching and reluctance to swallow.

CAUSES
Usually infection, and particularly by the feline viral rhinotracheitis virus (see page 179).

TREATMENT
Antibiotics will help if the infection is caused or aggravated by bacteria.

LICE

Like fleas, lice are wingless blood-sucking insects, but unlike fleas, they live attached to the hairs of the host. They live out their whole life cycle on the cat, sticking their eggs on to the hairs (visible as nits). They are not very common on cats.

SIGNS
Red, itchy spots on the skin, with excess scurf production
and sometimes bald patches caused by excessive grooming.
The adult lice and the nits are visible to the naked eye, but
the diagnosis can be confirmed by examining a hair sample
under the microscope.

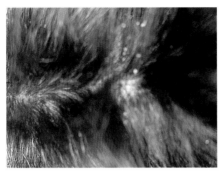

*Evidence of lice
infestation.*

CAUSES
It is usually caused by the feline biting louse, Felicola
subrostratus, although dog lice are also sometimes found on
cats. The adults can pass from one animal to another,
although they will only survive for a short time in the
environment.

TREATMENT
Insecticidal treatment needs to be used regularly for at least
four weeks, long enough to kill any eggs that may hatch out
during that time.

LIVER DISEASE
**The liver can be considered as the processing factory of
the body, playing an essential role in the cat's
metabolism. Because the cat is a pure carnivore, the
liver of the cat has lost the ability to carry out some of
the processes that other animals designed to cope with a
wider range of foods are able to manage, making the cat
particularly susceptible to the toxic effects of certain
substances.**

SIGNS
Liver disease tends to cause rather non-specific signs such
as lethargy, lack of appetite, vomiting, diarrhoea and weight
loss. More specific signs can include an enlargement of the
liver itself, and jaundice (see page 201).

CAUSES

There are many possible causes of liver disease, but the most important in the cat are:-

•Lymphocytic cholangitis: an inflammation of the liver that is thought to be caused by a disorder of the cat's immune system.

•Cholangiohepatitis: another form of liver inflammation most commonly caused by a bacterial infection that invades the bile ducts within the liver.

•Toxic hepatopathy: there are many poisons that can affect the liver of cats, including plants, household and garden chemicals, and drugs such as paracetamol. Quite a number of cats have died because their owners have dosed them with drugs not intended for use in that species.

•Hepatic lipoidosis: yet another strange-sounding liver disease of cats that can follow on from a period of starvation, or from other metabolic diseases such as diabetes mellitus (see page 161). Fat is laid down in the liver, causing serious interference with its normal function.

•Liver tumours: the liver is a common site for secondary tumours to settle that have spread from another site in the body, but it is also quite common for primary tumours to develop in the liver or in closely related structures such as the pancreas.

TREATMENT

Differentiating the various possible causes of liver disease in the cat can pose a considerable challenge to the veterinary surgeon. Blood tests, X-rays, and ultrasound of the liver may all be useful, but in some cases it is necessary to carry out a surgical biopsy, taking a small piece of liver tissue to be analysed under the microscope. Because the liver is important for breaking down many anaesthetics in the cat's body, and because blood clotting is often prolonged in affected animals, this procedure is not without significant risk. Nevertheless, this risk may well be outweighed by the benefit of obtaining a definitive diagnosis.

Once the cause has been established, steps can be taken to try and correct it, as well as providing supportive treatment for the cat. Fortunately, the liver has a good capability to regenerate, but if chronic liver disease is allowed to persist, the normal liver will become replaced by fibrous tissue, a process known as liver cirrhosis. Antibiotics are effective against liver infections, and corticosteroid drugs will help to control inflammatory problems. The surgical removal of tumours is only occasionally possible when an isolated non-malignant mass can be identified. Cats with liver disease need a low-fat, easily digestible diet, fed little and often. In severe cases, the cat may need to be hospitalised and fed via a fine tube passed down the nostril and into the stomach.

LUNG DISEASE

The lungs are a pair of organs surrounding the heart within the chest cavity and protected by the rib cage. A stethoscope can be used to listen to the sounds that the lungs make during respiration, and radiographs are very useful to 'look into' the chest for any abnormalities. An infection of the lungs is called pneumonia, and is not very common in cats, although it can develop as a complication of cat flu (see page 146). Like the liver, the lungs are also a very common site for secondary cancers that have spread from a primary tumour in other parts of the body. Other diseases affecting the lungs include pleurisy (page 219), lungworm (see below), haemothorax (page 190), pneumothorax (page 221), and diaphragmatic hernia (page 163).

LUNGWORM

Tiny parasitic worms that are swallowed with the cat's prey and live in the airways.

SIGNS
Infection with lungworms is very common in cats, but very often produces very little in the way of clinical signs. Severe lungworm infestations may cause coughing, and even secondary pneumonia and pleurisy, but this is rare.

CAUSES
The feline lungworm, Aleurostrongylus abstrusus, is usually passed on to cats via intermediate hosts such as rodents, and infection is therefore most common in young adult cats that enjoy hunting. The adults live in the lower airways of the lungs. The eggs that they produce develop into larvae which are then coughed up and passed out in the faeces to infect another host. A microscopic examination of the faeces may demonstrate the presence of these immature worms.

TREATMENT
Many cats recover without treatment, but a specific

worming preparation that is known to be active against this worm can be supplied by a veterinary surgeon if this problem is suspected.

LUXATING PATELLA
An instability of the kneecap that allows it to slip out of its normal position in the patellar groove on the femur (thigh bone).

SIGNS
Intermittent lameness, where the patella slips out of place and the affected hindlimb locks in position.

CAUSES
This can occur as a hereditary problem in pedigree cats, where the patellar groove does not form properly and the condition develops early on in life. It is much more common as a sequel to injury to the knee joint, where the ligaments that hold the patella in place tear and instability subsequently results.

TREATMENT
Mild cases may settle with rest, but there is a danger that long-term arthritis will develop if the condition is not rectified. An operation can be carried out to reshape the groove in the femur if necessary, and tighten the ligaments that hold the patella in place.

LYMPHOSARCOMA
A cancer of the lymphocytes – white blood cells that are found in the blood and lymphatic system. See cancer (page 143) and feline leukaemia virus (page 174).

M

MAD CAT DISEASE

See feline spongiform encephalopathy (FSE), page 176.

MASTITIS
An inflammation of the mammary glands.

SIGNS
One or more mammary glands of a lactating queen will become inflamed, producing signs of swelling, heat and pain. In severe cases, an abscess can form and burst. The queen usually becomes very depressed and off-colour. In some cases of chronic mastitis, the queen shows very little sign of problems at all, while the kittens develop gastrointestinal disturbances and die.

CAUSES
A bacterial infection of the mammary tissue.

TREATMENT
Hot poultices on the affected gland and antibiotic treatment will usually cure the condition, but it is essential that the kittens are removed and hand-reared to prevent further spread of infection via ingestion of the infected milk.

MEGAOESOPHAGUS
The oesophagus, or gullet, is the tube that carries the food from the mouth down to the stomach. In this condition, the muscular tube becomes weak and stretched, with food accumulating within it.

SIGNS
Regurgitation of a sausage of undigested food soon after eating. The cat will be very hungry, yet it will lose weight because a lot of the food it eats is not reaching the stomach.

CAUSES
Most commonly as a complication of feline dysautonomia (see page 171). Since this condition is becoming much less common, megaoesophagus is also being seen less

frequently. In rare cases, it is seen as a congenital problem in kittens.

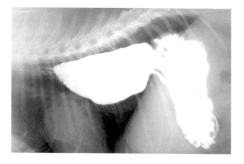

Dilated oesophagus, outlined by a barium swallow (white).

TREATMENT
Feeding small, semi-liquid meals with the cat eating in an upright position will help the food to pass down the oesophagus with the aid of gravity. Drugs can be used to try and stimulate the muscles to contract more effectively, but the long-term outlook is poor.

MELANOMA
A tumour of the pigment-producing cells within the skin.

SIGNS
Single lumps in the skin, usually darkly pigmented, that grow rapidly and have a strong tendency to spread to other parts of the body (see cancer, page 143).

CAUSES
In humans, it is known that excessive exposure to the sun can be a triggering factor. It is not thought that this is common in the cat.

TREATMENT
Surgical removal early on may be curative, but once the tumour spreads, the outlook is hopeless. Melanomas within the mouth carry a particularly poor prognosis.

MILIARY DERMATITIS
A term used to describe a skin condition where the cat develops multiple small scabs over its body, and especially along its back. See allergic dermatitis, page 126.

MITE INFESTATIONS

Mites are very small, eight-legged parasites, and there are several species that can cause problems in cats. Ear mites (see ear disease, page 166) are extremely common in young kittens, sometimes also causing a skin reaction around the head. Cheyletiella (see cheyletiellosis, page 148) is another surface-living mite that can cause skin problems. The demodectic mange mite is cigar-shaped and lives deep in the hair follicles, but is a very rare cause of skin disease in cats.

NASOPHARYNGEAL POLYPS

Strange polyps that can grow from the middle ear on a long stalk, down into the back of the throat, causing some obstruction to breathing and swallowing. See chronic rhinitis (page 149).

NEPHRITIS

An inflammation of the kidneys. See kidney disease (page 202).

NEPHROTIC SYNDROME

A less common form of kidney disease than chronic nephritis (see kidney disease, page 202).

SIGNS

The condition is most common in young male cats, and causes an accumulation of fluid under the skin of the limbs, the belly and sometimes within the chest.

CAUSES

The syndrome is due to an immune reaction within the body that damages the normal filtration system of the kidneys, allowing large amounts of protein to leak out of the blood and into the urine. Low protein levels then reduce the ability of the blood to draw fluid from the body tissues into the circulation, causing it to accumulate in abnormal sites around the body.

TREATMENT

Nephrotic syndrome is quite commonly associated with some degree of kidney failure, making management difficult because the high-protein diet needed to replace the excessive amounts being lost will aggravate the effects of renal failure. Diuretic drugs can be used to help remove excessive amounts of fluid, and anti-inflammatory treatment may help to control the underlying immune response that is causing the problem. Some cats with the condition can survive quite happily with treatment for several years.

NERVE INJURIES

These can commonly occur if a cat is involved in major trauma, such as a road traffic accident.

SIGNS
Lack of movement and sensation in the part of the body supplied by the particular nerve that has been damaged.

CAUSES
Bruising, or complete severance of a nerve.

TREATMENT
In the case of bruising, the affected nerve will quickly recover, but if a nerve has been severed, the loss of function will almost certainly be permanent. If this involves a major nerve to a limb or tail, amputation may be necessary (see amputation, page 129).

NUTRITIONAL IMBALANCES

Far more cats suffer from an excess of nutrients than from a deficiency in most Western countries (see obesity, page 216), but it is possible for cats to become ill if their diet does not contain the correct balance of minerals and vitamins. It must be stressed that although enough minerals and vitamins are a good thing, it is by no means true to say that more must be even better.

Nutritional imbalances seen in cats include:-

•Excess vitamin A – see hypervitaminosis A (page 197).
•Excess vitamin D is not common in cats, but it can be seen following the misuse of certain vitamin supplements, or due to poisoning with certain rodent baits. It causes calcium to be laid down in abnormal sites around the body.
•Taurine deficiency – a cause of heart disease (page 191) and blindness (page 138), that can be caused by feeding cats on a vegetarian diet. Some cats seem to have a higher requirement for this amino acid than others. At one time, many commercial cat foods did not have sufficient levels to supply the needs of all cats, but once this was realised, the content of all reputable brands was quickly adjusted.
•Thiamin deficiency – also known as vitamin B1, the vitamin is readily destroyed by heating, or by the presence of an enzyme called thiaminase found in certain species of

raw fish such as carp and herring. A deficiency initially causes depression and decreased appetite, but then develops on to severe neurological signs such as loss of balance, muscle weakness, loss of vision, and eventually collapse and death. Reputable proprietary diets have extra thiamin added to counteract the loss incurred during the cooking process.

• Calcium deficiency – see hyperparathyroidism (page 195).

• Vitamin E deficiency – see yellow fat disease (page 250).

• Essential fatty acid deficiency – cats have a more specific requirement for certain fatty acids in their diet than most other animals, and, again, can suffer from a deficiency if fed on a vegetarian diet. It has been associated with poor growth in young animals and poor coat condition.

OBESITY
An excessive accumulation of body fat.

SIGNS

You do not need a degree in veterinary science to recognise a fat cat! Fortunately, the cat is less likely to suffer from many of the problems such as coronary heat disease and strokes that make obesity such a health threat to humans, and arthritis and breathing disorders that are commonly aggravated by obesity in dogs. Indeed, most cats are much better able than their canine counterparts to regulate their food intake to match their requirements in the first place.

Fat cats are more likely to suffer from diabetes, and both arthritis and respiratory problems do occur, but cats are at less risk of suffering significant health problems as a result of being overweight than many other species. This is very fortunate – as it is also very difficult to manipulate the calorie intake of many cats, and especially those that are able to supplement their diet in the neighbourhood dustbin.

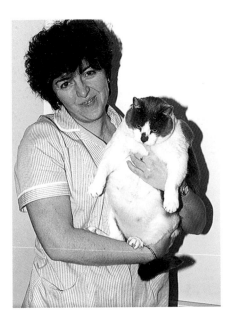

Obesity can lead to major health problems.

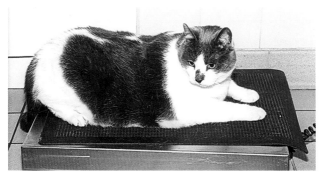

An obese cat should be put on a diet, and its weight should be monitored on a regular basis.

CAUSES

The cause of obesity is extremely simple: over a period of time the cat eats more calories than it burns up. It is very easy to blame this upon 'hormones', and it is certainly true to say that neutered cats are more likely to put on weight than entire ones, but obesity in cats is only very infrequently due to any hormonal imbalance that requires medical treatment. However, it is important to differentiate between a cat that may look fat because it has a swollen abdomen, and one that is genuinely overweight, because the former can be a sign of several serious diseases. Feeling the covering of fat over the bones of the spine may help to distinguish the two.

TREATMENT

Care has to be taken in trying to force a cat to follow a new diet, as, unlike dogs, cats really will starve themselves until their health is threatened, such as by hepatic lipoidosis (see liver disease, page 206). Prevention is always better than cure, so weigh your cat regularly and pick up any increase in weight early on, as minor changes to the diet at that stage will prevent problems from developing.

Dry cat foods are convenient and help to exercise your cat's teeth, but most of them are very dense in calories and will fool the cat's innate ability to regulate its energy intake. The key to preventing obesity is to feed a balanced cat food with an energy content that is matched to its requirements. Once a cat has become significantly overweight, special prescription diets are available that can be gradually introduced into the feeding regime in place of the higher calorie foods. Your veterinary surgeon is the best person to advise you on the correct diet for your cat and to monitor any weight reduction programme.

OSTEOMYELITIS
An infection of the bone.

SIGNS
If a limb is affected, it will cause lameness, tenderness and warmth over the site of the infection. The cat may well be off-colour and run a temperature. Sometimes infection can establish itself in other bones, such as within the vertebrae of the spine, where it will cause signs related to pressure upon the spinal cord. See spinal disease, page 237.

CAUSES
Infection may be introduced directly into the bone, such as by a deep penetrating bite-wound or a complicated fracture that breaks the skin, or the infection may spread in the bloodstream from some other site in the body, such as an abscess, and then settle in one or more bones.

TREATMENT
The condition can be diagnosed with X-rays, and, if open to the surface, a swab can be taken and cultured in a laboratory to confirm that bacteria are present, and to test which antibiotics are likely to be most effective. Several weeks of antibiotic treatment are often needed to clear a bone infection thoroughly.

OSTEOSARCOMA
A particularly malignant form of bone cancer (see cancer, page 143). If it occurs on a limb bone it can sometimes be cured by prompt amputation.

OTITIS
An inflammation of the ear, that can either take the form of otitis externa, affecting the outer ear, or otitis media and interna, that affects the middle and inner ears below the ear drum. See ear disease, page 166.

OTODECTIC MANGE
Ear mite infestation – see mite infestation (page 212) and ear disease (page 166).

PANCREATITIS

An inflammation of the pancreas, which is situated just below the stomach and is responsible for producing digestive enzymes and insulin, the hormone that controls glucose levels in the blood.

SIGNS

May be acute, or more commonly in cats, chronic. Acute pancreatitis causes severe abdominal pain and vomiting, whereas the chronic form of the disease causes vague non-specific signs such as loss of appetite, weight loss and depression. A blood test and abdominal X-rays will help to diagnose the problem, although sometimes an exploratory operation is necessary.

CAUSES

The cause is not known.

TREATMENT

Acute cases need intensive treatment with intravenous fluids and pain-killing drugs. Some affected cats go on to develop long-term digestive problems or diabetes mellitus due to permanent damage to the organ. A bland low-fat diet will help in cases of chronic pancreatitis.

PANSTEATITIS

See yellow fat disease, page 250.

PARALYSIS

See nerve injuries (page 214) and spinal disease (page 237).

PLEURISY

The pleural cavity is a potential space that lies between the lungs and the wall of the chest. It is normally only filled with a very small amount of fluid, but can, quite commonly, fill with abnormal amounts of varying types of secretion.

SIGNS
Laboured breathing and lethargy. Cats may also go off their food and lose weight.

CAUSES
The most common causes of a build-up of fluid in the pleural cavity are:-

•Heart disease – see cardiomyopathy (page 145).
•Tumours – especially lymphosarcoma (see cancer, page 143), a cancer of the white blood cells that, in young cats, quite commonly affects the mediastinum – the connective tissue that surrounds the heart and divides off the two sides of the chest.
•Infection – the build-up of pus around the lungs is called pyothorax. The source of the infection is often unknown, and may spread from a distant site within the bloodstream rather than directly from a penetrating wound into the chest.
•Feline infectious peritonitis (see page 172) – the 'wet' form of this disease can often cause an accumulation of pale-yellow coloured fluid in the pleural cavity.
•Diaphragmatic hernia (see page 163) – a cat may slowly adjust to the initial breathing difficulties caused by the interference with chest function that a tear in the diaphragm causes – to the point that the condition may go undiagnosed. If a part of the liver, which lies just below the diaphragm, slips up into the chest cavity, this can cause an accumulation of fluid and renewed breathing problems.

As can be seen from the above list, sorting out the cause of 'fluid on the chest' can be quite difficult. A blood test may help to differentiate between some of the conditions, but a chest X-ray is usually necessary, plus an analysis of some fluid that is drawn off. Ultrasound may also be useful in examining affected cats, particularly in the case of heart disease. Handling a cat with severely compromised breathing, and particularly administering a sedative or anaesthetic, can be quite a risky procedure, but it is usually necessary in order to try to identify the cause of the problem.

TREATMENT
Drawing off the accumulated fluid will result in improved breathing, but unless the cause is treated, more will quickly accumulate. Long-term diuretic treatment will help with cases of cardiomyopathy, but in the case of FIP, little can be done. The long-term outlook for cats with chest tumours is

Drawing fluid from an anaesthetised cat with pleural effusion.

also poor, but some will respond well to chemotherapy, giving at least a useful extension of life, if not a cure.

A tear in the diaphragm can be corrected surgically, and a bacterial infection can often be treated successfully, although this may involve repeated draining off of pus and infusion of antibiotics directly into the pleural cavity, as well as orally.

PNEUMONIA
An infection of the lung tissue. See lung disease (page 208).

PNEUMOTHORAX
The presence of free air in the chest cavity.

SIGNS
Rapid, shallow breathing and increasing distress as the cat struggles to get its breath.

CAUSES
Most commonly caused by an accident that produces chest damage and allows air to leak from the lungs. It can be diagnosed radiographically.

TREATMENT
In mild cases the leak will heal over and air will be reabsorbed, but more severe cases may require a chest drain.

POISONING
Although cats are generally much more fastidious about what they will eat than dogs, and so are less likely to ingest poisons, they are also much less able to detoxify

certain poisonous substances within their body, and so may have a severe reaction to a product that may be relatively harmless in other species.

There are many hundreds of substances that can be poisonous to cats – even water can be toxic if taken in sufficiently large quantities! The most important ones are outlined below, but the following general principles should be borne in mind:–

Many cases of poisoning in cats are accidentally caused by their owners. Never give your cat any medicine that has been prescribed for another species of animal (including humans) unless you have cleared it with your vet first.

Speed is essential when dealing with a case of suspected poisoning. Unless the substance is caustic (very unlikely with cats), you should try to make the cat vomit while it is still in the stomach, by dosing the cat with a small crystal of old-fashioned washing soda, or a strong solution of salt water. However, do not delay unnecessarily trying to administer an emetic, as the vet may well need to wash out the stomach under an anaesthetic.

Keep any relevant information about the nature of the poison, such as the packet in the case of pesticides, and contact your vet without delay. If your cat has contaminated its coat with a harmful substance, physically prevent it from grooming itself, preferably by wrapping its body and legs in a towel, until it has been thoroughly cleaned.

CAUSES/TREATMENT

RODENTICIDES
These are quite a common cause of poisoning, sometimes ingested indirectly by a cat catching and eating a rodent that has been slowed down by eating poisoned bait. Some, such as warfarin, act by interfering with blood clotting, causing death by internal bleeding. Others, such as the mouse bait alphachloralose, and strychnine, which is only allowed to be used under licence to control moles, affect primarily the nervous system. Vitamin K injections can be given to counteract the anticoagulant poisons.

INSECTICIDES
Poisoning by this group of compounds generally occurs in cats when proprietary insecticide preparations have been

mis-used, resulting in overdosing. This most commonly occurs with the organophosphorus group of insecticides such as dichlorvos, found in many sprays and flea collars, and is particularly seen if a cat that is wearing an insecticidal collar is also treated with a topical preparation. Always read the instructions on products thoroughly and follow them closely. Signs of poisoning include excessive salivation, vomiting, diarrhoea, muscle twitching, and eventually convulsions and death. These signs can be reversed if treated early with injections of the antidote, atropine.

MOLLUSCICIDES
Slug bait, usually containing metaldehyde, is one of the commonest causes of poisoning in cats, as many pets seem to be attracted to ingesting it. The effects are similar to those caused by organophosphorus poisoning, but there is no specific treatment other than trying to reduce the absorption of the bait, and drugs to control its toxic effects.

MEDICAL PREPARATIONS
Aspirin, paracetamol, aminoceptophen, and ibuprofen (sold as Nurofen) are all examples of drugs that are sold over the counter for use in humans, yet potentially very toxic to cats, even in quite small doses. The toxic effects vary with the drug concerned, and specific antidotes only exist in a few cases.

DISINFECTANTS AND PRESERVATIVES
Cats are very susceptible to the toxic effects of coal tar derivatives such as phenolic disinfectants, fungicides such as PCP and wood preservatives such as creosote. There have been cases reported of cats dying as a result of using bedding made from wood shavings treated with these types

Feet contaminated with tar.

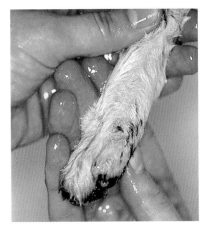

Cleaning the feet with swarfega.

of drugs, or from cats rubbing along treated wood and then swallowing the preservative when they try to groom it off. Even disinfectants that are considered safe for human use may be much more toxic to cats, and will usually be ingested if applied to the skin. Poisoning results in excessive salivation, abdominal pain, weakness, convulsions and eventually death. There are no specific antidotes.

PLANTS

Many plants that are found in the house and garden can be harmful to cats, and indoor cats do often seem to wish to chew on some form of vegetable matter – providing a pot of grass growing on a window ledge may provide an acceptable alternative. Laurel, ivy, philodendron, laburnum,

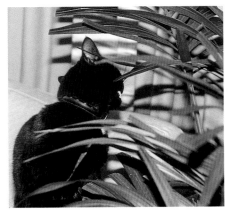

Some house plants an be harmful to cats.

poinsettia, and the pine needles from Christmas trees, as well as many others, have been reported as causing toxic reactions in cats. In mild cases this may involve no more than a digestive upset or a sore mouth, but the effects can be more severe. It is best to play safe and remove any houseplants out of reach if cats are spotted chewing on them.

PYOTHORAX
A build-up of pus in the chest. See pleurisy (page).

PYOMETRA
An infection of the womb that results in a build-up of pus within the uterus.

SIGNS
This problem is obviously only seen in entire females (although sometimes a 'stump pyometra' can develop in the end of the womb that is left in place after the spaying operation). If the cervix remains closed, the womb will fill up with pus, distending the abdomen, and the cat will show signs of illness related to the toxins released into the body, such as lethargy, an increased thirst and sometimes vomiting. If the cervix opens, a thick, smelly vulval discharge will be seen.

CAUSES
The condition often starts as chronic endometritis, a thickening of the lining of the womb that results from a hormonal imbalance and is a common cause of a failure to reproduce (see infertility, page 198).

TREATMENT
Antibiotics alone are not likely to clear the condition, and surgical removal of the womb and ovaries is necessary.

PYREXIA
Not a disease, but a clinical sign, pyrexia means an abnormally elevated body temperature, or fever. The normal body temperature in the cat is around 101.5 degrees Fahrenheit (38.6 Centigrade). 'Pyrexia of unknown origin' or PUO, is the term used when a cat is running a temperature but the cause cannot be determined.

SIGNS
Lassitude, lack of appetite, and an elevated rectal temperature. Some owners may be aware that their cat feels hotter than normal.

CAUSES
Infections are the most common cause, including bacterial infections as a result of fights, viral infections such as feline leukaemia virus (page 174) or protozoan infections such as feline infectious anaemia (page 171). Feline infectious peritonitis (page 172) can cause pyrexia, which is particularly difficult to diagnose, as the blood test for the disease is notoriously unreliable.

However, pyrexia is not always a sign of infection and may also be caused by autoimmune reactions (see anaemia page 131) and tumours (see cancer, page 143).

Care must be taken in interpreting an elevated temperature, as the figures quoted above are only averages, and, by definition, some cats will have a higher than average body temperature as their normal temperature. Stress and exercise may also elevate the reading obtained.

TREATMENT
The underlying cause must be determined and, if possible, treated. Antibiotics will only be of value if the cause is a bacterial infection.

Q FEVER

A disease that cats are commonly exposed to, but that rarely causes illness. It can cause problems in humans, but affected cats are not thought to be a likely source of infection.

SIGNS
Usually none, but there is a suggestion that it may cause abortion (see abortion page 123).

CAUSES
A tiny micro-organism called Coxiella burnetti.

TREATMENT
Difficult with drug treatment alone, but surgical removal of the lesions will often result in a cure.

RABIES

Rabies is a deadly disease of the nervous system caused by a tiny, bullet-shaped virus. It is thought to be able to infect any warm-blooded animal, but some species are more susceptible than others – cats being moderately so. The UK and several other European countries such as Iceland, The Netherlands, Spain, Eire and Portugal are free of the disease.

SIGNS
The initial stage of rabies in the cat is characterised by quite subtle behavioural changes, which progress on to the furious phase, where the cat becomes uncontrollably aggressive and can readily pass on the virus to other animals by biting. Paralysis usually develops, first in the extremity that was originally bitten, and eventually spreading to the whole body, resulting in coma and death.

In areas where rabies is known to be present, the brain of suspect cases will always be examined by a laboratory to check for the disease. Any animal that develops clinical signs of rabies will almost certainly die from the disease, but preventative injections can be given to humans after exposure to the virus.

CAUSES
The main reservoir of the disease in Central Europe are foxes. Great efforts are being made to reduce the incidence of the problem by dropping bait, dosed with oral vaccine, to protect them in the wild. In Asia, South America and Africa the dog acts as the principal reservoir of disease, whereas in North America skunks and racoons harbour the virus.

PREVENTION
Cats as well as humans can be protected from the disease by vaccination, although the use of rabies vaccine in the UK is currently restricted only to animals that are due to be

exported. At the present time, the UK maintains its rabies-free status by a six-month quarantine period that applies to any cat that is imported into the country. The only exception to this is for commercially traded cats and dogs, born and kept isolated in registered premises in the European Community and meeting certain strict criteria.

There is strong pressure for relaxation of these regulations to allow the movement of cats within the European Community and from rabies-free countries if they are permanently identified with an injectable microchip, are vaccinated against rabies, and are subsequently blood-tested to ensure the vaccine has taken properly.

RETAINED TESTICLES

The testicles of the male cat begin life within the abdomen, close to the kidney, and soon after birth migrate down the inguinal canal in the groin and into the scrotum. This is important, because in order to be able to produce sperm, they have to be kept slightly below normal body temperature. In some cats, the testicles fail to descend normally, and are retained within the abdomen. If one testicle is involved, the condition is called monorchidism; if neither are present in the scrotum, it is known as cryptorchidism.

SIGNS
The absence of one or both testicles in the scrotum is very obvious as the cat matures. If the testicle fails to desend, it may twist upon itself, cutting off its blood supply and becoming gangrenous internally, or develop into a tumour later on in life.

CAUSES
The condition is believed to be hereditary.

TREATMENT
The retained testicle(s) should be surgically removed, not only because of the risk of complications, and to prevent a cat with a hereditary defect from breeding and passing on the problem to future generations, but also because, although the retained testicle will not produce sperm, it will produce male hormones. A cryptorchid cat, or a monorchid that has had one normal testicle removed, will therefore look like a castrated male but retain all the physical and behavioural characteristics of a tom cat.

RINGWORM

Q: When is a worm not a worm?
A: When it's a ringworm.
Despite its confusing name, ringworm is a fungal infection of the skin, but it is a name far more easily remembered than its medical term, dermatophytosis.

SIGNS
Patches of hair loss, typically growing outwards in an expanding circle, redness and scaling of the skin. It is more common in young cats, and most often affects the hair around the head, ears and forelegs. Some long, fine-haired cats such as the Persian may carry the fungus on their coat without showing any signs of skin disease.

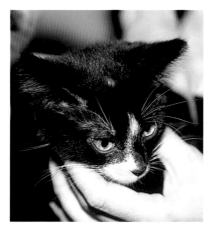

Evidence of ringworm.

The characteristic sign of ringworm on a human.

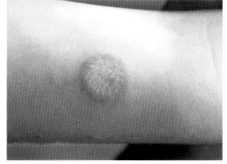

CAUSES
There are many different fungi that can cause ringworm, but by far the commonest in the cat is Microsporum canis,

officially the dog ringworm, but actually far more frequently found on cats. The fungus does not actually affect the skin, but grows on the hairs. It can sometimes be seen to fluoresce under a special ultraviolet lamp called a Woods Light, and the fungal spores may be seen if hairs are examined under a microscope. However, the most reliable test for ringworm infection is to culture a hair sample on a special medium, although it can take up to three weeks to get a result.

TREATMENT
Hair clipping and anti-fungal washes will help to control the problem, but the most effective cure is a course of treatment with a drug called griseofulvin, which has to be given for several weeks to allow it to grow into the hair and so protect it against infection. Hygiene is very important, as the spores are very resistant, and can be transmitted via bedding or grooming implements as well as direct contact.

Ringworm can cause skin disease in humans; so if your cat is diagnosed as suffering from the problem, it is essential to wash hands thoroughly after handling the cat and to seek medical advice if any unusual skin lesions develop.

RODENT ULCER
A form of eosinophilic granuloma on the lip (see eosinophilic granuloma complex page 169).

ROUNDWORM
A very common parasite that lives in the small intestine of the cat. The dog roundworm has been implicated in causing a disease known as visceral larval migrans in humans, where the larvae of the worm enter the body and cause a reaction. In very rare cases, this can cause damage to the eyesight, especially in children. Although it is theoretically possible for the cat roundworm to cause this problem in humans as well, they are not thought to be a significant source of human infection.

SIGNS
A heavy infestation with roundworms, especially in kittens, may cause loss of condition, diarrhoea, and a bloated appearance to the belly. It is very common for cats to harbour the worms without showing any signs of disease, shedding eggs into the faeces. As the eggs are only visible under the microscope, owners may only become aware that

their pet has roundworms if a worm is vomited up or passed in the faeces.

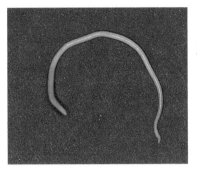

Roundworm.

CAUSES
There are two species of roundworm that affect the cat, Toxocara cati, which is the most common, and Toxocara leonina. The adult worms are up to six inches (15cms) long and string-like, living in the intestine and absorbing the nutrients that they need from the bowel of their host. The eggs are passed in the faeces and ingested by earthworms, beetles, rodents or birds, and then reinfect another cat when they eat one of these animals. It is also possible for immature worms to pass through the mammary tissue into the milk, and thus infect kittens while they are still suckling from their mother.

TREATMENT
Kittens should be routinely treated for roundworms from eight weeks of age, and adults should also be treated a couple of times a year. The most effective preparations are available from your veterinary surgery, where you will also be able to obtain advice on the best regime for your cat. Worming preparations are now available in tablet, powder and liquid form.

SALMONELLOSIS

The Salmonella group of bacteria is a common cause of severe food poisoning in humans and many species of animals. Its particular significance is the fact that cats infected with the organism may pass it on to humans.

SIGNS
Acute diarrhoea, sometimes with vomiting. The cat is often unwell and runs a temperature.

CAUSES
Infection may be contracted by eating contaminated food, particularly raw or partially cooked meat. It is also possible for cats to contract it from other animals or humans in the household.

TREATMENT
Culture of the cat's faeces in the laboratory is the only sure way of diagnosing the condition, but any cat that has severe gastrointestinal signs and is unwell should receive veterinary attention. Strict hygienic precautions should be observed with such cats, cleaning the litter tray thoroughly with disinfectant, washing hands regularly after handling the cat, and keeping them away from food preparation areas. Animals that are recovering from the infection may remain carriers of the organism for a considerable length of time.

SARCOMA

A malignant tumour of the connective tissues. The precise name will depend upon the type of connective tissue involved, such as osteosarcoma, which describes a malignant tumour of the bone (see cancer, page 143).

SEBORRHOEA

This is an abnormality in the secretion of sebum, or natural oils, on to the coat from sebaceous glands in the skin.

SIGNS
It can take two forms: seborrhoea oleosa, an over-production of oil that causes a greasiness of the skin and coat; and seborrhoea sicca. The latter is much more common, and causes a dry scaliness of the skin due to an underproduction of sebum.

CAUSES
It usually develops secondarily to some other skin condition, such as a parasitic infection with fleas or mites, fungal infections, or metabolic disorders caused by problems such as liver disease. Nutritional imbalance is another important cause, and some cats do not seem to be able to absorb the fatty acids that they need in their diet as well as other cats.

TREATMENT
The underlying cause must be removed if possible. Anti-seborrhoeic shampoos can be used in cats, although human anti-dandruff products should not be used without veterinary advice as many of them contain coal tar products that can be toxic to cats when licked off. A veterinary supplement of evening primrose oil given on a daily long-term basis can often be very helpful in controlling this problem.

SEPTICAEMIA
Blood poisoning – or illness due to the presence of harmful bacteria in the bloodstream.

SIGNS
This is potentially a very serious condition, and the cat is likely to be running a temperature and to be severely off-colour. In advanced cases, the toxins released by the multiplying bacteria can cause septic shock (see shock, page 235) and organ collapse.

CAUSES
Bacteria may enter the bloodstream through several possible routes, such as from infected teeth or gums, or any penetrating wound. Most commonly, it follows from a bite wound that has resulted from two cats fighting.

TREATMENT
This condition will usually respond well to antibiotics once a diagnosis has been made, although it is useful if a blood

sample is sent to a laboratory to confirm the diagnosis, and to ensure that the antibiotic being used is effective against the organisms causing the problem.

SHOCK

Circulatory collapse, with inadequate blood supply to essential body organs.

SIGNS
Weakness, rapid pulse, pale mucous membranes (such as the lining of the mouth), shallow breathing and cold extremities.

CAUSES
Many different causes, such as blood or fluid loss, heart failure, major allergic reactions and serious infections. Reduction of the blood supply to vital organs causes damage to those organs, which, in turn, makes the shock worse. This can rapidly prove fatal unless treated promptly and aggressively.

TREATMENT
First-aid treatment of shock involves stemming any significant blood loss and keeping the patient comfortably warm until professional assistance can be obtained. Intensive veterinary treatment is needed to reverse shock, centering on the administration of large volumes of intravenous fluids to restore the circulating blood volume. Drugs, such as large doses of corticosteroids and vasodilators to open up the blood supply to the tissues, are of value in some cases.

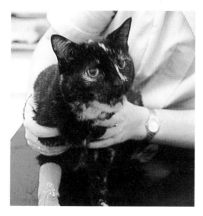

Intravenous fluids may need to be administered via a drip when a cat is suffering from shock.

SKIN CANCER
See cancer (page 143), melanoma (page 211), and solar dermatitis (below).

SKIN DISEASE
The cat has relatively few ways in which its skin responds to disease, and many different disease problems look very similar. Clinical signs are mainly due to the effects of self-inflicted trauma caused by the cat over-grooming with its very rough tongue. This most commonly takes the form of bald patches, where the hair is worn away as it attempts to grow, or miliary dermatitis, with small papules on various sites around the body, and especially along the back.

CAUSES
The major causes of skin disease in the cat can be seen under their relevant entries:-
•Allergic dermatitis (page 126): far and away the most common.
•Skin parasites: see fleas (page 181), cheyletiellosis (page 148), and lice (page 205).
•Ringworm (page 230).
•Pyoderma: bacterial skin infection that develops secondarily to some other cause.
•Seborrhoea (page 233).
•Acne (page 125).
•Skin tumours: some benign and others malignant (see cancer, page 143).
•Hormonal hair loss: see alopecia (page 128).
•Solar dermatitis (see below).
•Cowpox (page 155).
•Eosinophilic granuloma complex (page 169).

SINUSITIS
See chronic rhinitis, page 149.

SOLAR DERMATITIS
Sunburn of the skin due to the effects of ultraviolet radiation on unpigmented skin that is not protected by a heavy growth of hair.

SIGNS
Reddening and crusting of the ear-tips and nose of white-

coated cats. Long-standing cases can progress to squamous cell carcinoma, a form of skin growth (see cancer, page 143).

CAUSES
Repeated exposure to ultra-violet radiation in summer.

TREATMENT
The only really effective treatment is to keep the cat indoors while the sun is at its highest. Tattooing of the affected areas has been tried to help protect the skin with pigment, and non-toxic titanium dioxide based sun-block cream can be applied, but most cats will promptly remove it.

SPINAL DISEASE
The bony vertebral column plays a vital role in locomotion, and protects the fragile spinal cord that carries nervous impulses from the brain around the body. Any damage to the spine can have very serious consequences and lead to permanent paralysis.

SIGNS
Disorders of the cervical spine (neck) will affect all four limbs, whereas disorders of the lumbar spine (back) will only affect the hindlimbs. Pain, weakness, or complete paralysis of the limbs can result, depending upon the degree of damage.

CAUSES
'Slipped discs' are not nearly as common in the cat as in dogs and humans, but osteomyelitis can sometimes develop within the vertebrae or the intervertebral discs and cause similar signs. Most spinal problems in cats occur as a result of trauma, particularly due to road traffic accidents.

TREATMENT
Bruising of the spinal cord, or very minor fractures of the vertebrae will heal with strict rest, but more severe fractures may require major surgery to stabilise them. If the spinal cord has been damaged, immediate surgery to remove the pressure on it may be successful, but the outlook is very guarded. A cat with permanent paralysis of its hindlimbs, and certainly of all four limbs, should be euthanised for humanitarian reasons.

STOMATITIS

An inflammation of the oral cavity. See gingivitis, (page 187).

STROKES

See ataxia, page 136.

STUD TAIL

'Blackheads', or plugged hair follicles, on the skin of the tail. See acne, page 125.

SUNBURN

See solar dermatitis, page 236.

TAPEWORM

As its name suggests, the tapeworm is a long, flat parasite that lives in the small intestine of the cat. It buries its head into the lining of the bowel, holding on with suckers and hooks. Its body can be up to twenty inches (50cms) in length, and is divided into segments along its length. The end segments develop into sacs full of eggs, called proglottids. These proglottids are passed out from the rectum, and then burst open to release the eggs.

SIGNS
Tapeworm infestations may cause intestinal discomfort, itchiness around the anal area and weight loss, but very often they cause no signs of illness at all. Owners may well notice the segments either in the faeces, or stuck to the hair around the anus, and although they are harmless to humans, most owners find them disturbing.

CAUSES
There are two species of tapeworm that commonly affect the cat, and their life cycles are very different. The most common is Dipylidium caninum, and in order to complete its life cycle, the eggs have to be eaten by flea larvae. The disease is passed on to another host when it eats an infected flea while grooming itself.

The other species is Taenia taeniaeformis, and its eggs

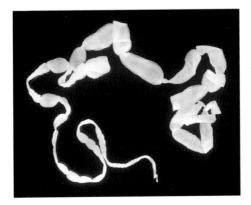

Tapeworm.

239

have to be ingested by a small mammals such as mice, voles, rats and squirrels. The life-cycle is then completed if an infected animal is caught and eaten by a cat. Therefore, Dipylidium caninum infestation will only occur in cats that have come into contact with fleas, and Taenia taeniaeformis is only found in cats that hunt and eat wild animals.

TREATMENT
Cestocides, which are drugs specifically active against tapeworm, are widely available, and it is important that an owner either uses a combination wormer that is effective against both tapeworm and roundworm, or clearly establishes the cause of their own cat's problem. Although old-fashioned all-in-one wormers needed an extended course of treatment, modern veterinary preparations are available that are highly effective against both types of worm in just a single dose. Injectable cestocides can also be administered by vets to cats that will not allow their owners to give drugs orally. It is essential to take steps to eradicate fleas both on the cat and in its environment in order to prevent re-infestation, and cats that hunt wildlife may need to be treated for tapeworm on a regular basis.

TETANUS
Tetanus in cats is a very uncommon condition, as they are very resistant to the disease, but cases are occasionally seen.

SIGNS
Stiffness of the limbs and contraction of the facial muscles, giving the affected animal a surprised look, which may progress to collapse and spasms of the muscles, and eventually death.

CAUSES
Clostridium tetani is a bacterium that is commonly found in the soil, and causes tetanus by proliferating in a deep, contaminated wound and releasing toxins into the body.

TREATMENT
Surgically cleaning all dead tissue from the original wound, and prompt treatment with high doses of penicillin will cure the condition in its early stages, but intensive supportive treatment is required if a cat with more advanced signs is to survive.

TETRAPLEGIA

Paralysis of all four limbs, usually caused by a severe spinal injury in the neck region. See spinal disease (page 237).

THIAMINE DEFICIENCY

Thiamine is a B vitamin that is essential to life, but is normally present in ample quantities in a meat-based diet.

SIGNS
Cats become off-colour and refuse food. Their gait becomes uncoordinated and the muscles stiff. Convulsions may develop in advanced cases.

CAUSES
Thiamine is destroyed by prolonged cooking, and although this is compensated for in commercially available diets, a deficiency can develop in cats fed on home-prepared thoroughly cooked meat. Fish contains an enzyme that breaks down the vitamin, and cats fed on a diet consisting mainly of raw fish may also develop the problem.

TREATMENT
Correction of the diet and injections of thiamine can cure the problem quickly in its early stages, but the outlook is poor once advanced brain damage has been caused.

THIRD EYELID PROTRUSION

Cats have upper and lower eyelids, but unlike humans, they have a third eyelid that quickly moves across from the inner corner of the eye to protect it from impending injury.

SIGNS
In a cat suffering from this condition, the third eyelid of one (or both) eyes will protrude across the eye, partially obstructing the cat's vision. Cats also suffer from a specific syndrome, whereby they are generally perfectly healthy but have protruding third eyelids and often mild but chronic diarrhoea.

CAUSES
Damage to the nerve that controls the third eyelid will cause it to protrude, such as with Horner's syndrome (page 194)

and feline dysautonomia (page 171). It has recently been discovered that a virus known as a torovirus can infect the cat and cause the signs of a protruding third eyelid and chronic diarrhoea.

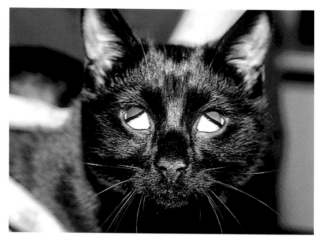

Third eyelid prolapse.

TREATMENT
There is very little that can be done to treat this condition, but if the cause is a viral infection, owners can be reassured that it always does correct itself after about three weeks. Symptomatic treatment can be used for the diarrhoea, and ensuring the cat is getting a good balance of minerals and vitamins will help to boost its resistance to fight off the infection.

THROMBOSIS
See iliac thrombosis, page 198.

THYROID DISEASE
See hyperthyroidism, page 195.

TICKS
Ticks are wingless, parasitic insects that bury their mouthparts into the skin of their host, gripping firmly while they fill their bodies with a massive meal of blood.

SIGNS

A tick first appears as a small grey, white or cream coloured dot, attached to the skin, and gradually grows over a few days to look like a large wart – although close examination will reveal the legs of the insect close to the skin. They sometimes cause some local irritation, but do not generally cause their hosts too much discomfort. In some parts of the world, tropical ticks may play a significant role in transmitting disease (see Q fever, page 227).

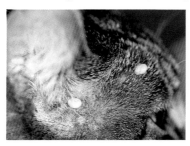

Ticks seen on cat's head.   *Close-up of a tick.*

CAUSES

The tick only feeds once in a year, and when it has filled its body with a store of blood, it drops off and lays its eggs on the ground. These hatch out into tiny seed ticks, which climb up on to plants such as long blades of grass and wait patiently for the next meal to walk by. Cats therefore tend to pick them up mainly around the head, as they brush through the grass. The commonest species of tick found on cats in the UK is Ixodes ricinus, which is normally found on sheep and cattle, but they are very non-specific about their hosts, and even animals such as hedgehogs may carry them into suburban gardens.

TREATMENT

The thing not to do with a tick is to yank it off while it is still alive, because this will be painful for the cat and carry a considerable risk of leaving the mouthparts buried in the skin, which can then cause quite a severe reaction to develop. The tick should be killed, and the simplest way to do this is by spraying it directly with an insecticide designed to kill fleas. It will then shrivel up over about 24 hours, and will either fall off by itself or it can be picked off without any resistance.

243

TOXOPLASMOSIS

This single-celled parasite is commonly found in the cat. Although it only infrequently causes serious disease in the cat, it is of particular relevance because of the possibility of infection being passed from cats to humans, where it can occasionally cause serious problems to pregnant women and young children.

SIGNS

The majority of cats that are exposed to the parasite quickly develop an immune response to it, showing no significant signs of illness other than mild diarrhoea, and becoming resistant to further infection. Disease problems are most likely in young cats, or those whose immune system has been suppressed by infection with an agent such as feline immunodeficiency virus, or by certain types of drug treatment. In these animals it can cause lethargy, loss of appetite and fever. It may also affect the lungs, causing pneumonia, damage to the liver, and to the central nervous system, causing incoordination, behavioural disorders and blindness.

A blood test will determine whether a cat has antibodies to the organism. However, two tests, two to three weeks apart, are needed to distinguish between a cat that is actively infected, and one that has been exposed in the past and is now immune. In the former case the levels of antibodies will be rising significantly, whereas in the latter they will be steady. In severe cases of toxoplasmosis, the cat may die before antibodies can be measured in its blood, and the diagnosis has to be made on the basis of a post mortem examination.

CAUSES

The disease is caused by the protozoan parasite Toxoplasma gondii, which lives within the body tissues and its eggs are shed in the faeces of infected cats, remaining infectious for up to a year in moist soil. They are then ingested by any one of a wide range of intermediate hosts, such as earthworms and insects, and then into other hosts such birds or rodents, and then back to cats again. They may also be taken in by grazing ruminants, and are an important cause of disease, especially in sheep.

Although they can affect any species of mammal or bird, the cat is thought to play a crucial role in its life cycle. The disease in humans is much more common in countries where raw or undercooked meat is traditionally eaten, and it is thought that this demonstrates that contaminated food is the main source of infection in humans rather than cats.

TREATMENT
A combination of drugs can be used to treat the problem in cats once a diagnosis has been made, although mild cases will be self-limiting anyway. The main problem is how to control the spread of the disease from cats to humans. It should be remembered that Toxoplasma gondii is probably the commonest parasite in the world, and yet clinical disease in either cats or humans is not widespread because of the ability of the immune system to control it under normal circumstances. However, infection can, and does, cause severe developmental abnormalities in new-born babies, and therefore careful consideration should be given to the steps that can be taken to control its spread. The Toxoplasmosis Trust, a British organisation set up to promote information about the disease, recommends the following steps for pregnant women or those particularly at risk:-

•Only eat meat that has been thoroughly cooked.
•Wash your hands and cooking utensils after preparing raw meat.
•Wash fruit and vegetables thoroughly to remove all traces of soil.
•Clean out litter trays daily, using rubber gloves, or get someone else to do it.
•Use gloves when gardening and wash hands afterwards.
•Cover children's outdoor sandboxes to prevent cats using them.
•Consult your vet if your cat is unwell.

ULCER
A break in the skin or mucous membrane that can be caused by physical injury or infection. See eosinophilic granuloma complex (page 169), calicivirus (page 142), and corneal ulceration (page 153).

UMBILICAL HERNIA
See hernia, page 193.

URINARY TRACT DISEASES
See kidney disease (page 202), feline urological syndrome (page 177).

UVEITIS
An inflammation of the iris and associated structures within the eye.

SIGNS
A painful and inflamed eye, with contraction of the pupil and change in colour of the iris that surrounds it.

CAUSES
Uveitis is often associated with severe injury to the eye, or to some other underlying disease, such as toxoplasmosis (page 244), feline infectious peritonitis (page 172), and feline leukaemia virus (page 174). In some cases, no underlying cause can be identified.

TREATMENT
Mydriatics, drugs that relax and dilate the pupil, are very useful in relieving the pain associated with this condition, and reducing the chances of long-term complications developing. Anti-inflammatory drugs will also help. Sometimes the condition becomes recurrent, with repeated attacks occurring over an extended period.

VAGINAL DISCHARGE
See pyometra, page 225.

VOMITING
Carnivores such as cats are able to vomit quite readily to eject indigestible food from their body. This is sometimes done to feed their young.

SIGNS
True vomiting of food from the stomach should be distinguished from the more passive act of regurgitation, where undigested food is brought back up, often almost as a sausage, as regurgitation is more likely to relate to a problem with the oesophagus or stomach (see, for example, megaoesophagus page 210), rather than one further down the digestive tract.

CAUSES
Causes of vomiting include:-

•Gastroenteritis: an inflammation of the digestive tract (see diarrhoea, page 163)
•Specific infections: their importance is uncertain, but an organism called Heliobacter has been found in the stomach wall of cats that suffer from vomiting. This organism is also credited with being a major cause of gastric ulcers in humans, and the possibility exists that it could be passed from cats to humans.
•Food sensitivity: some cats seem unable to digest certain foods, and the first line of treatment for a cat that is otherwise healthy but throws up with some regularity is to try a change to a bland, low-fat diet. Milk may also cause a problem. Some cats also seem to be prone to vomiting after eating dry food, especially if a large amount is eaten quickly.
•Systemic disease: due to toxins that build up in the body with conditions such as liver disease (page 206) and kidney disease (page 202).
•Foreign bodies: less common than in dogs due to their more fastidious eating habits, but, nevertheless, a wide

247

range of unusual objects have been surgically removed from the stomach of cats, including needles on the end of lengths of cotton that have been ingested by kittens. While an object lodged in the stomach may cause irritation and subsequent vomiting, one that passes further down the digestive tract and becomes obstructed in the small intestine will also cause severe vomiting due to a 'damming back' effect.

•Constipation (see page 153).

•Poisoning (see page 221).

•Tumours: fortunately, stomach cancer is rare in the cat.

•Pyloric stenosis: usually a problem of young cats (especially Siamese kittens), this condition is caused by an abnormality in the pyloric sphincter, a group of muscles which control the passage of food out from the stomach into the intestine. If this fails to open properly, the cat will suffer from projectile vomiting, where food is very violently ejected from the stomach.

DIAGNOSIS/TREATMENT

Cats with persistent vomiting need to have further investigations carried out to identify the cause. A blood test can rule out underlying systemic disease, and X-rays are very useful for highlighting disorders in the digestive tract. Sometimes the problem can be seen on a plain X-ray, but it is often necessary to administer a contrast medium, such as barium, and to take multiple pictures as it travels out from the stomach and into the intestines.

Endoscopy, where fibre-optics allow direct examination of the wall of the stomach down a special viewing tube, is available in some specialist centres, and some procedures such as the removal of small foreign bodies can even be carried out non-invasively by this means.

WARFARIN POISONING

One of the commonest forms of poisoning in the cat due to ingestion of rat poison (see poisoning, page 221).

SIGNS
Generally relate to abnormal bleeding in various sites around the body, and include bloody diarrhoea, weakness, pale mucous membranes, lameness due to bleeding into the joints, and sometimes small areas of haemorrhage visible under the mucous membranes. Death can occur due to blood loss (see haemorrhage, page 189).

CAUSES
Small doses of poison often have more effect than one large dose, and can even be taken in indirectly by eating rodents that have been poisoned. The active ingredient interferes with the action of Vitamin K in the body, which is essential for the normal blood-clotting mechanism.

TREATMENT
It is essential that cats with suspected warfarin poisoning are handled very gently to avoid further bruising and blood loss. A blood test can confirm the diagnosis, but treatment with the specific antidote, vitamin K injections, will usually be given as a safety precaution even before the diagnosis has been confirmed. In cases of severe blood loss, blood transfusion may be necessary as a life-saving measure.

WOUNDS
See abscesses (page 124), haemorrhage (page 189), first aid and nursing (page 90).

XYZ

XANTHOMATOSIS
A fairly rare condition involving the laying down of abnormal deposits of fatty material around the body.

SIGNS
The most obvious sign of the condition is multiple skin lesions around the body, consisting of single or multiple nodules that may ulcerate.

CAUSES
Disease such as diabetes mellitus, that affect the metabolism of fat within the body, may cause the problem to develop, but it can also be hereditary.

TREATMENT
The lesions will resolve on their own if the high blood fat levels can be reduced by tackling the underlying problem.

YELLOW FAT DISEASE
An inflamation of the fatty tissue under the skin.

SIGNS
Loss of appetite, depression, tenderness over the body, and sometimes the cat will run a temperature.

CAUSES
It is caused by a deficiency of vitamin E in the diet. This has been associated with the feeding of high levels of fish, particularly red tuna.

TREATMENT
Correction of the diet, sometimes with anti-inflammatory drugs.

ZOONOSES
This is the term used to describe diseases that are transmissible from animals to man. The health risks from a responsibly kept pet cat are very slight indeed. The

following are feline diseases that sometimes cause problems to their humans. More details can be found under their specific headings :-

Cat scratch Fever (page 147)
Cheyletiellosis (page 148)
Chlamydiosis (page 148)
Cowpox (page 155)
Heliobacter: see under vomiting (page 247).
Fleas (page 181)
Rabies – not in the UK (page 228)
Ringworm (page 230)
Salmonellosis (page 233)
Toxoplasmosis (page 244).

INDEX